Dr Sarah Brewer
natural
health
guru

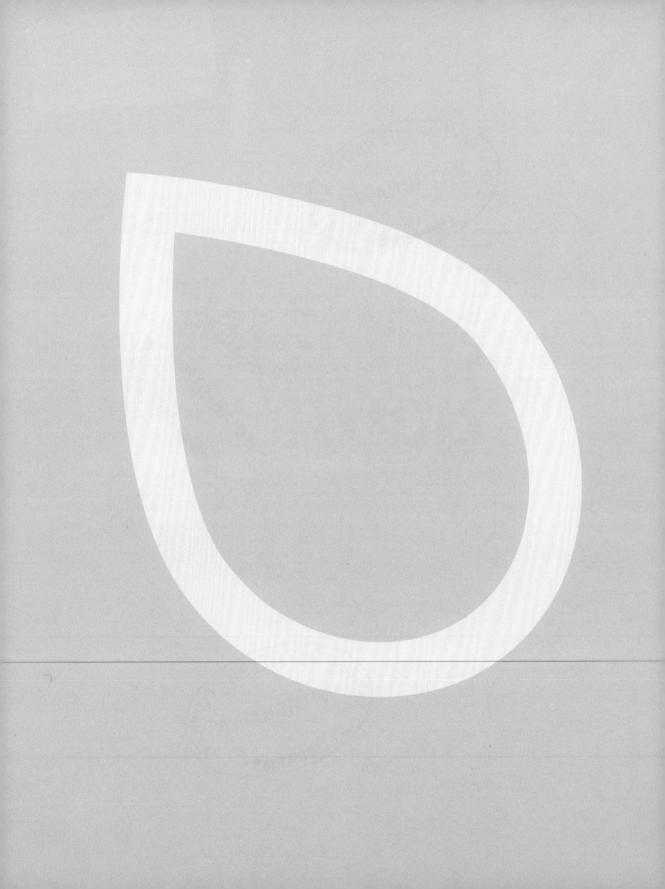

overcoming
asthma

the complete complementary health program

Dr Sarah Brewer

In association with The Complementary Medical Association

DUNCAN BAIRD PUBLISHERS
LONDON

Natural Health Guru: Overcoming Asthma
Dr Sarah Brewer

For my wonderful husband, Richard

First published in the United Kingdom and Ireland in 2009 by
Duncan Baird Publishers Ltd
Sixth Floor
Castle House
75–76 Wells Street
London W1T 3QH

Conceived, created and designed by
Duncan Baird Publishers

Copyright © Duncan Baird Publishers 2009
Text copyright © Dr Sarah Brewer 2009
Artwork copyright © Duncan Baird Publishers
Photography copyright © Duncan Baird Publishers

Managing Editor: Grace Cheetham
Editor: Kesta Desmond
Managing Designer: Manisha Patel
Designer: Gail Jones
Commissioned artwork: Mark Watkinson
Commissioned photography: Simon Smith and Toby Scott
Styling: Mari Mererid Willliams
Picture research: Susannah Stone

British Library Cataloguing-in-Publication Data:
A CIP record for this book is available from the British Library

ISBN: 978-1-84483-765-6
10 9 8 7 6 5 4 3 2 1

Typeset in Univers
Colour reproduction by Scanhouse, Malaysia
Printed in China by Imago

Publisher's note:
The information in this book is not intended as a substitute for
professional medical advice and treatment. If you are pregnant
or are suffering from any medical conditions or health problems,
it is recommended that you consult a medical professional before
following any of the advice or practices suggested in this book.
Duncan Baird Publishers, or any other persons who have been
involved in working on this publication, cannot accept responsibility
for any injuries or damage incurred as a result of following the information, exercises or therapeutic techniques contained in this book.

Notes on the recipes:
Unless otherwise stated: use medium eggs, fruit and vegetables.
Use fresh ingredients, including herbs. Do not mix metric and
imperial measurements.
1tsp = 5ml, 1tbsp = 15ml, 1 cup = 250ml

contents

overcoming asthma
introduction

The word "asthma" comes from a Greek word, *aazein*, meaning "to breathe out with an open mouth" or "to pant". Although everyone suffers from breathlessness from time to time, someone with asthma experiences recurrent shortness of breath, chest tightness and wheezing that's often worse at night, first thing in the morning and after exercise.

Asthma can develop at any age, but it usually starts during the first few years of life – one in four children with asthma develop symptoms before their first birthday. Although many children "grow out" of asthma during their teens, a recent US study found that wheezing continued during adolescence in more than half (58 percent), especially in those who were overweight, or who started puberty early. But, even if symptoms disappear during adolescence, they often return in later life. According to a study from New Zealand, up to a third of children whose asthma had gone by the age of 18 developed renewed symptoms by the age of 26. Just as worryingly, researchers found that nine percent of participants who developed the condition by age 26 had never had asthma as children.

The number of people with asthma is increasing and has at least doubled over the last 25 years. In some countries, such as Australia, an estimated one in four children, one in seven adolescents and one in 10 adults are affected. The number of asthma attacks experienced by those with asthma is also increasing, and is now six times higher in children and three to four times higher in adults compared with 25 years ago.

The exact reason why asthma is becoming more common remains unknown, but is believed to result from interactions between our immune system and our 21st-century diet, lifestyle and environment. According to experts, the four most likely culprits are:

- Increased exposure to indoor allergens such as house dust mites and cockroaches as a result of modern housing conditions and because we spend more time indoors.
- Over-cleanliness and over-use of antibiotics, which reduce our exposure to the bacteria that prime our immune system against over-zealous allergic reactions.
- Obesity and lack of physical activity, which promote inflammatory reactions and reduce lung fitness.
- Our changing Western diet – our increasing consumption of omega-6 vegetable oils promotes inflammation; and we eat too little antioxidant-rich fruit, vegetables, probiotic bacteria, and anti-inflammatory omega-3-rich fish oils.

Follow your doctor's advice

The information and advice given in this book is for general information only. It is not intended to replace individual advice from your own doctor. This book takes a holistic approach, and is designed to complement the treatments your doctor prescribes. It is intended to act as a guide only. Always follow the advice of your doctor or other healthcare professionals who know your individual needs in detail. In particular, never stop taking your asthma medication unless you are stepping down your treatment according to the personal asthma management plan that your doctor has worked out with you (see page 20).

You can use this information to your advantage by reducing your exposure to indoor allergens, losing any excess weight, exercising regularly, and following a more healthy diet and lifestyle. This book will tell you how to succeed in all of these things.

The ideal goal for everyone with asthma is to lead a symptom-free life, with no compromises made as a result of their condition. Children in particular should be involved in normal play, including full participation in exercise and sport. As long as the diagnosis is made, optimal treatment is prescribed, drugs are taken correctly and dietary and lifestyle changes are made to reduce triggers and improve immune function, a symptom-free life is possible. Unfortunately, however, many people with asthma accept waking at night wheezing, coughing and feeling breathless – they shouldn't! Nocturnal symptoms and recurrent shortness of breath after exercise are signs that your treatment is failing – something that you can change.

This book provides the information you need to overcome your asthma symptoms. It informs you about the important dietary and lifestyle changes you can make, why regular exercise is so important, the benefits of breath control and relaxation; and other complementary approaches that will help you.

Everyone is different and no diet and lifestyle plan will suit all individuals. For this reason, I've drawn up three different approaches: a gentle, moderate and full-strength program, one of which is likely to suit you. To help you work out which program is right for you, follow the detailed questionnaire on pages 75–76.

For most people, the gentle program is a good place to start. This introduces you to healthy eating principles, such as cooking without salt, eating more fruit, vegetables and fish, and eating less red meat. I suggest taking food supplements at the lowest doses shown to have a significant, beneficial effect on asthma symptoms. I also show you some useful

Look out for these symbols
Throughout this book I have included boxes that highlight useful, interesting or important pieces of information. Each box bears a symbol (see below). The arrow symbol indicates that a box contains practical instructions. The plus sign means that the box contains additional information about the subject being discussed or about asthma in general. The exclamation mark indicates a warning or a caution.

breathing exercises and introduce you to approaches such as aromatherapy and homeopathy.

If your questionnaire answers reveal a likely sensitivity to dietary sulfites, the moderate program will help you to exclude sulfites from your diet as much as possible. I suggest you take food supplements at higher doses, and I show you a more intensive breath control regime based on the world-renowned Buteyko method. I also introduce you to complementary approaches such as reflexology and meditation.

If your questionnaire answers point to a likely sensitivity to aspirin, the full-strength program provides an eating plan that significantly reduces your exposure to dietary salicylates (see pages 48–49). I suggest food supplement doses at the higher end of the therapeutic range, and introduce you to complementary techniques such as acupressure and acupuncture.

Updated information, new recipes and the latest research findings will be added regularly to my website www.naturalhealthguru.co.uk. Visit regularly to tell me how you get on with the programs. Good luck!

Understanding asthma

In this section I describe the nature of asthma and its **causes, triggers, signs and symptoms**. I explain how asthma is diagnosed, and the **range of treatments that your doctor may prescribe**. Asthma tends to be a relapsing and remitting condition, which means there are times when your symptoms are troublesome – for example, when you catch a cold – and times when they're not. Your doctor should give you a **personal management plan** that means you can step up your treatment when your asthma plays up, and step it down when your symptoms go away. The important thing to remember is that **asthma is associated with long-term inflammation** in your lungs. So even when your symptoms are relatively well controlled, your airways may still be red and inflamed. You can help to **monitor what's happening in your lungs** by using a peak flow meter – this measures how well air is flowing through your airways at any one time. If you notice your peak flow readings are falling, this is a sign that you may soon experience asthma symptoms – and that it's time to step up your treatment. On the following pages I explain **how to use a peak flow meter** and **how to assess the readings**. I've also provided a **six-step action plan** describing what you should do during an asthma attack.

what is asthma?

Asthma is a long-term, inflammatory condition that affects the lungs. It varies considerably in severity. In mild cases you may notice only a slight cough. In severe cases, it may be so difficult to breathe that you can't get enough oxygen into your bloodstream and you lose consciousness. To understand what goes wrong in asthma, it's helpful to know something about the anatomy of the lungs and how breathing works.

The healthy respiratory system

Every time you inhale, air passes through your mouth or nose, along a tube called the trachea and into your upper chest. From here it goes into your left and right bronchi. Each bronchus enters one lung and divides more than 20 times to form smaller and smaller branches known as bronchioles. These are smaller than a millimetre in diameter and are surrounded by a thin layer of muscle that can constrict or dilate.

The bronchioles lead into grape-like clusters of air spaces called alveoli, of which you have more than 300 million. These tiny alveoli are about the size of the full-stop at the end of this sentence. They give the internal surfaces of your lungs a total area that's roughly the size of a tennis court. Oxygen diffuses across the thin walls of the alveoli into the network of tiny blood vessels (capillaries) that surround them. Every minute, your heart pumps five litres (175fl oz) of blood through these tiny capillaries. Within the capillaries, oxygen binds to the red blood pigment, hemoglobin, in exchange for the waste gas carbon dioxide, which diffuses back into the alveoli ready for you to exhale. Oxygen is then carried in your blood to tissues and organs all over your body.

The lining of the lungs The bronchi and bronchioles have a special lining called the respiratory epithelium. This contains "goblet" cells that secrete mucus and a watery fluid – these keep your airways moist and trap inhaled particles such as pollen, dust and bacteria. The respiratory epithelium also contains tiny, hair-like projections known as cilia. The cilia beat in a co-ordinated fashion to move mucus and trapped particles up out of your lungs on the so-called "ciliary escalator". This keeps your lungs clean by bringing up mucus that you get rid of by coughing or swallowing. Ciliary activity is inhibited by several noxious agents, including smoking. The smoke from a single cigarette immobilizes the ciliary escalator for several hours.

What happens in asthma

If you have asthma, your lung airways become red, inflamed and overly sensitive. The underlying cause of this inflammation varies from person to person (see

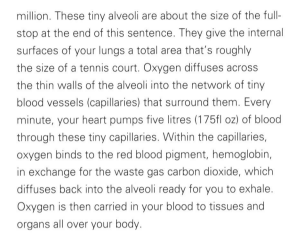

The amount of air you breathe
Altogether, your lungs can hold an average of three litres (105fl oz) of air at any one time. Every minute of every day, you breathe in around four litres (140fl oz) of fresh air, at rest. During heavy exercise, the amount of air you breathe in and out can increase by as much as 20 times. The air you inhale contains 21 percent oxygen but just 0.03 percent carbon dioxide. The rest is mostly inert nitrogen gas.

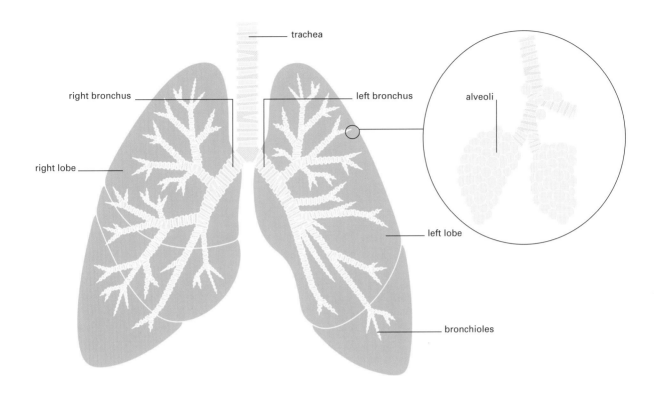

trachea

right bronchus

left bronchus

alveoli

right lobe

left lobe

bronchioles

pages 12–13). The specific triggers of an asthma attack can also vary. Examples of triggers include exercise, heightened emotion, viruses, allergens and cold air. These make the irritated airways go into spasm and become constricted. When the airways constrict, your chest wall muscles have to work harder to get air in and out of your lungs.

During an asthma attack your chest feels tight and you become increasingly short of breath (known as dyspnea). Breathing out becomes especially difficult, and the turbulent air flow through your narrow airways produces an audible wheeze. If the attack progresses, the lining of the airways swells and produces excess mucus – this often results in a further bout of tightness and wheezing six to eight hours after the initial attack. In severe cases, airway narrowing and plugs of mucus can block the flow of oxygen into the lungs. Air flow

The healthy lungs

Your lungs are two sponge-like organs situated within your chest. Air passes along your trachea and enters your lungs via your bronchi. From here it passes into tiny air passages known as bronchioles. These lead to balloon-like sacs called alveoli – where oxygen passes into your blood.

becomes so impaired that wheezing stops, too little oxygen reaches the body, and waste carbon dioxide gas builds up. This is a life-threatening situation.

The narrowing of the airways that occurs in asthma is usually reversible with medication. But, even between attacks when you are symptom-free, your airways may still be red and inflamed. Asthma treatment aims to damp down the underlying inflammation so that attacks of breathlessness, wheezing or coughing do not recur.

causes and triggers of asthma

There appear to be two different types of asthma: allergic and non-allergic. Each type is associated with different causes and triggers. A "cause" is linked to why you have developed asthma. A "trigger" is something that sets off an individual attack.

Causes of allergic asthma

Allergic asthma tends to begin in childhood and improves with age. It is linked with hayfever, eczema and a family history of allergies.

Genes A combination of genes can be passed from parent to child that increases the chance of developing allergic conditions such as asthma, eczema and hayfever. This allergic tendency is called "atopy". The child of one parent or both parents with asthma is twice as likely to develop asthma as the child of parents without asthma.

Birth weight Bigger babies (weighing over 7lb/3.2kg at birth) may be at higher risk of developing allergic asthma, especially if they have large heads and long bodies. The exact reason is unknown, but it may be linked with good nutrition in the first six months of pregnancy, followed by poor nutrition in the last three. This is thought to affect the way part of the immune system, known as the thymus gland, develops.

Bottle-feeding Babies who are introduced to milk other than breast milk before four months are 25 percent more likely to develop asthma and 40 percent more likely to develop a wheeze than those who are exclusively breastfed.

Overcleanliness A child's home environment is also important: over-cleanliness, which reduces exposure to bacteria, may prevent a child's immune system developing properly. Repeated exposure to dirt and childhood infections is believed to be healthy in that it may prime an immature immune system to become less sensitive to common allergens. Research shows that young children attending nursery or preschool groups from the ages of two or three seem less susceptible to developing asthma.

Causes of non-allergic asthma

Non-allergic asthma tends to begin in adult life. There is often no family history of allergy, and sufferers often have sinusitis, nasal inflammation and nasal polyps.

Weight A man with a waistline of more than 102cm (40in) and a woman with a waistline greater than 88cm (35in) are five times more likely to have non-allergic asthma than those of normal weight.

Cigarette smoke Exposure to cigarette smoke at any age increases the risk of non-allergic asthma. A baby exposed to passive smoking is up to three times more likely to wheeze than one reared in a smoke-free environment. Newly diagnosed adults with asthma are more likely to be current or ex-smokers than never-smokers, with women smokers at the greatest risk.

Gender Until the age of 11, asthma is more common in boys than girls. After puberty, the pattern changes so more girls develop wheezing while symptoms in boys improve. By adulthood, two out of three people with asthma are female. Older women who take oestrogen as part of hormone replacement therapy (HRT) are also more likely to develop asthma than those not taking oestrogen.

What triggers an attack?

The triggers for an asthma attack can be divided into two categories: allergens, such as pollen and dust mites; and non-allergens, such as emotion and exercise. If you have allergic asthma, the following allergens may be responsible for triggering an attack.

- Pollen – proteins in the pollen from grasses and trees can trigger asthma in some people, especially during thundery weather (because the humidity of a thunderstorm causes pollen grains to break up; then pollen granules are spread by stormy air currents).
- Moulds – poor housing associated with water leaks and dampness promotes the growth of moulds, whose airborne spores can trigger asthma.
- House dust mites feed on dead skin cells found in household dust and bedding. Their digestive enzymes and fecal matter contain proteins to which many people develop an allergic reaction. Asthma symptoms that appear all year round are often linked with house-dust-mite allergy.
- Food and food additives (see pages 42–55).
- Insect venom – the injected venom of bees, wasps, hornets and ants contains more than 100 chemicals that can trigger an allergic reaction in some people.
- Nuts – a nut allergy is a sensitivity to nut proteins. The most common nut allergen is peanut, but many sufferers are also sensitive to other nuts, such as walnut, almond, pistachio, hazelnut and cashew.

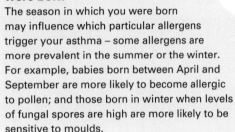

The season in which you were born
The season in which you were born may influence which particular allergens trigger your asthma – some allergens are more prevalent in the summer or the winter. For example, babies born between April and September are more likely to become allergic to pollen; and those born in winter when levels of fungal spores are high are more likely to be sensitive to moulds.

- Latex – rubber is a common trigger of asthma, especially in healthcare workers who are sensitive to powdered natural rubber latex gloves.

If you have non-allergic asthma, your asthma attacks are not triggered by allergens. Instead, any of the following may be responsible.

- Exercise.
- Cold air.
- Atmospheric pollution.
- Household chemical sprays.
- Medications – aspirin, ibuprofen and betablockers can trigger an asthma attack in some people.
- Cigarette smoke.
- Viral infections – in children, eight out of 10 asthma attacks are linked with respiratory viral infections that sensitize the airways to other triggers.
- Respiratory sensitizers – chemicals that irritate the airways, such as chlorine.
- Emotions – strong emotions such as over-excitement, anger, hilarity and stress can trigger asthma in some people.
- Acid reflux – acid moving from the stomach into the oesophagus can trigger an asthma attack.

signs and symptoms

Asthma can occur at any age. Untreated asthma causes recurrent attacks of coughing, wheezing, tightness in the chest and shortness of breath. Symptoms are often worse during the night and with exercise, but their severity and duration are highly variable and unpredictable.

Early warning signs of an asthma attack

Some people with asthma are able to spot the early warning signs that an attack is impending. If you can recognize early clues, you can take treatment that may help to prevent an attack coming on. The early warning signs of asthma are unique to each person and may vary from attack to attack. Sometimes people close to you may become familiar with the warning signs and can alert you.

Look for any of these signs and ask people close to you to be aware of them, too: dark circles under the eyes; heavy, watery or glazed eyes; changes in breathing; dry mouth; coughing; excessive mucus that may seem thicker or more watery than normal; headache; itching around the mouth or throat; nasal congestion; pallor; palpitations or a racing pulse; reduced ability to exercise; sleeping difficulties; sneezing; sweatiness; feverishness; tiredness; exhaustion; and weakness. You may also feel a general sense of slowing down or restlessness, or wanting to be left alone. People around you may notice that you become unusually quiet, moody, or over-excitable.

Checking your peak flow reading (see pages 16–17) is also a useful early warning sign as there is usually a downward trend in peak flow numbers before an asthma attack.

Signs and symptoms of an asthma attack

Asthma attacks vary in severity. During a mild attack you may cough, wheeze and feel some tightness in your chest. If symptoms progress and become more severe, you need urgent medical treatment. These are the signs and symptoms of a severe asthma attack:

- Severe coughing, wheezing, shortness of breath and tightness in the chest.

Symptoms that appear at work

If you notice that your asthma symptoms are worse during working hours or appear for the first time when you start a new job, you may have occupational asthma. You may also notice that you get relief from symptoms during weekends and holidays. Sometimes occupational asthma may cause delayed symptoms that appear at the end of a day at work, and that go away after a prolonged break. Occupational asthma is caused by exposure to specific substances at work. This is different to "work-aggravated asthma", which describes pre-existing asthma that is made worse by non-specific dust and fumes at work. The commonest work-related asthma triggers are cold air (for example, in storage rooms), dust (especially in old buildings) and manual labour. Cigarette smoke is also a trigger. If you think your asthma symptoms are related to your work, ask your doctor, asthma nurse or occupational health department at work for advice. You may be eligible for compensation in some countries.

- Inability to walk far owing to shortness of breath.
- Breathing that is shallow, and either faster or slower than usual.
- Difficulty talking or concentrating.
- Hunched shoulders.
- Nasal flaring.
- Retraction (pulling back) of flesh above your sternum and collar bones, and between and below your ribs when struggling for breath.
- A grey/bluish tinge to your lips and the skin around the mouth and fingernails (owing to lack of oxygen).
- Severely reduced peak flow numbers (usually below 50 percent of your personal best; see page 17).

Swollen airways during an asthma attack
Air normally flows freely through the bronchi, but during an asthma attack the muscles of the bronchi contract, the inner lining becomes swollen and inflamed, and mucus builds up. The restricted air flow makes breathing difficult.

Can children grow out of asthma?
Although many children grow out of asthma during their teens, more than half experience wheezing during adolescence – especially those who are overweight, or those who start puberty early. In one study of seven-year-olds with asthma, 20 percent no longer experienced asthma by age 14, and 40 percent no longer had symptoms by age 42. The prognosis is better the earlier the asthma starts. One study suggests that two-thirds of all children who wheeze before the age of three no longer have symptoms by the age of six unless they have an allergic tendency and also have eczema and hayfever. Children whose symptoms are more severe or frequent in childhood are also more likely to continue wheezing into adult life. Even if asthma appears to go away, there is no guarantee that it will stay away. Overall, boys are more likely to grow out of asthma than girls.

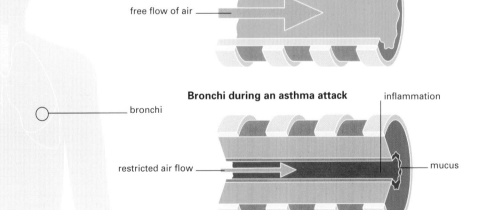

bronchi

Normal bronchi

free flow of air

Bronchi during an asthma attack

inflammation

restricted air flow

mucus

diagnosing and monitoring asthma

A doctor diagnoses asthma on the basis of your symptoms and by examining you. Once you've been diagnosed with asthma it's important to monitor how well it is controlled from day to day.

Diagnosing asthma

Your doctor will ask you about your symptoms – and when they occur – and about any family history of allergies. He or she will look at your chest for any signs that breathing requires more work, listen to your chest for wheezing and ask you to blow into a peak flow meter. Other signs of asthma are tachypnea (rapid breathing) and tachycardia (rapid heart rate).

Diagnosing asthma in the under fives Asthma is suspected in any child with recurrent wheezing and coughing, shortness of breath, or noisy breathing. If the diagnosis is in doubt, a doctor may prescribe a drug to dilate the airways (a bronchodilator; see pages 18–19) to see if this helps (although bronchodilators aren't always effective in young children).

Monitoring asthma

Once you've been diagnosed, you'll need to use a peak flow meter to monitor how well your lungs are working. This is a device that shows how fast you can blow out and therefore how constricted your airways are. When you are well, your airways are relaxed and your peak flow readings are high; but when your asthma is uncontrolled, your airways narrow and your peak flow readings are low. To use a peak flow meter:

- Move the marker to the lowest position on the scale (not necessarily zero).
- While standing, inhale deeply. Put the mouthpiece between your teeth and seal your lips around it.
- Blow into the meter as hard and as fast as you can.
- Take the peak flow meter out of your mouth and check how far the marker has moved along the numbered scale. Make a note of this number.
- Move the marker back to its lowest position and repeat the test twice more. Your reading is the best of these three results.

It's a good idea to record your peak flow several times a day (plot the results on a graph), especially if your asthma is not well controlled. It's also important to know your "personal best" peak flow number. You can get this by measuring your peak flow twice a day for two to three weeks when your asthma is under good control – your personal best is the highest reading. This helps you assess how well your asthma is controlled at any one time (see chart opposite). If your peak flow is in the green zone, your asthma is under control; if it's in the yellow zone, your lungs are inflamed (take action – see pages 20–21); if it's in the red or "danger" zone, seek immediate treatment.

Nitrous oxide test Another way to monitor your asthma involves a relatively new device that measures the amount of nitric oxide (NO) in the air you exhale. The higher the level of NO, the more inflammation is present in your lungs.

Assessing how well your asthma is controlled

if your personal best peak flow reading is:	you are in the green zone if your peak flow reading is:	you are in the yellow zone if your reading is between:	you are in the red zone if your peak flow reading is:
100	above 80	80 and 50	below 50
125	above 100	100 and 63	below 63
150	above 120	120 and 75	below 75
175	above 140	140 and 88	below 88
200	above 160	160 and 100	below 100
225	above 180	180 and 113	below 113
250	above 200	200 and 125	below 125
275	above 220	220 and 138	below 138
300	above 240	240 and 150	below 150
325	above 260	260 and 163	below 163
350	above 280	280 and 175	below 175
375	above 300	300 and 188	below 188
400	above 320	320 and 200	below 200
425	above 340	340 and 213	below 213
450	above 360	360 and 225	below 225
475	above 380	380 and 238	below 238
500	above 400	400 and 250	below 250
525	above 420	420 and 263	below 263
550	above 440	440 and 275	below 275
575	above 460	460 and 288	below 288
600	above 480	480 and 300	below 300

treating asthma

The aim of asthma treatment is the total control of your symptoms so you can enjoy normal activities in your daily life. You're likely to be prescribed two drugs: a preventer and a reliever. If these don't control your asthma, there are additional drugs that can help. Your doctor will also work with you to devise a personal asthma management plan so you are confident about how to deal with any worsening in your symptoms.

Preventers and relievers

You inhale preventers and relievers directly into your lungs using inhaler devices. This is why asthma drugs are often simply referred to as "inhalers" or "puffers".

Preventers These are corticosteroid drugs, such as beclometasone or fluticasone, that damp down inflammation in your lungs. They prevent asthma attacks if taken regularly, but when inflammation is severe, they may take up to 14 days to produce a noticeable effect. Preventers are used every day – even when you don't have symptoms. Unfortunately, because preventers don't produce the same instant relief as relievers, it's estimated that one in two people with asthma don't use them as prescribed. This is a great shame – you can't control your asthma unless you control the underlying inflammation first. Preventer inhalers are usually white, orange, red or brown. You will normally be prescribed a preventer inhaler if:

- You have breathlessness, coughing attacks, wheezing or tightness three or more times a week.
- You need to use your reliever inhaler more than twice a week.

- You have disturbed sleep owing to coughing or chest tightness once or more a week.
- You have asthma symptoms when you develop a chest infection or are exposed to cigarette smoke.

Relievers These are drugs such as salbutamol or terbutaline. They are designed for use when you experience asthma symptoms. They work by relaxing smooth muscles in your airways so your bronchioles dilate. This quickly makes breathing easier, and the effects last from three to six hours. However, relievers can only relax your airways – they do not tackle the underlying inflammation that leads to asthma in the first place. Because of this, if you need to use your reliever inhaler regularly – more than twice a week – you should ideally use a preventer inhaler every day. Reliever inhalers are usually blue or green.

Delivery systems The most common way to take preventers and relievers is via a metered-dose inhaler. This contains the treatment drug either in a suspension that you shake before use or in a solution (no shaking required). The inhaler delivers a set dose of drug that you inhale into your lungs (I recommend you have your inhaling technique checked regularly by a nurse or doctor). The other ways to take preventers and relievers are as follows:

- Spacers – these were originally designed for use by young children. They hold a cloud of drug that can be inhaled up to 10 seconds after activating the device.
- Nebulizers – these are used during severe

asthma attacks. They vaporize the drug so it can be breathed into the lungs more easily, usually through a mask.

- Breath-actuated devices – these are easier to use than a standard metered-dose inhaler because the act of breathing in triggers the device.

Additional asthma drugs

If both a reliever and the regular use of a preventer drug at a high dose don't control your symptoms, you may be prescribed further drugs – these are sometimes referred to as "add-ons".

Protectors This is sometimes known as a "long-acting reliever"; it's used when you still suffer from nocturnal or exercise-induced symptoms despite treatment with a preventer. Protector drugs include salmeterol and formoterol, which are similar to reliever drugs, but have a slower onset of action and help to keep airways open for up to 12 hours. You will need to use all of your inhalers together – the preventer, the protector, plus the reliever when necessary. You should not use a protector without a preventer.

Leukotriene receptor antagonist This is another add-on drug. It damps down inflammation by reducing the production, or activity, of inflammatory chemicals released by immune cells. Regular use can improve lung function, reduce the sensitivity of the airways, improve nasal congestion in patients also suffering from allergic rhinitis, and allow the dose of inhaled corticosteroids to be reduced or sometimes withdrawn.

Cromone This type of drug, which includes cromoglicate and nedocromil, helps asthma by reducing the allergic response to inhaled allergens such as pollen. It prevents the release of immune chemicals such as histamine from immune cells.

What to do if you have an attack

Take your reliever treatment immediately, preferably with a spacer.

Sit down – don't lie flat – and try to relax.

Wait five to 10 minutes. If your symptoms disappear, you don't need to do anything else.

If your symptoms continue, call your doctor or, if breathing is difficult, call an ambulance.

Continue taking your reliever inhaler (preferably with a spacer) every few minutes until help arrives.

If you go to hospital, take your asthma treatments (or details of their names and dosages) with you.

Immunotherapy

You may be offered immunotherapy to treat asthma. This is designed for allergic asthma and is most effective if your asthma results from a strong allergic reaction to a single airborne allergen. The treatment is also known as hyposensitization or desensitization – it re-trains your immune system to no longer react to airborne allergens such as pollen, moulds or house dust mites.

During immunotherapy you are given a series of skin-prick tests in which an extract of a suspected allegen is pricked into your skin. Initially, very dilute doses are used so as not to trigger a reaction. The concentration is then slowly increased at each weekly injection to help your immune system gradually adapt to the offending substance. When you eventually reach a dose that would normally trigger symptoms, treatment is kept at that dose and given every two to four weeks. Doses may need to be stepped down and then increased again if you start to get a reaction. A word of caution: receive immunotherapy injections only from a qualified doctor experienced in the technique. There is a risk of a severe allergic reaction (anaphylaxis) or a severe asthma attack if the build-up phase of treatment is progressed too quickly or procedures are not followed properly.

Some immunotherapists place drops under your tongue rather than using injections. Clinical trials suggest this is effective in treating allergic rhinitis and reducing the onset of asthma. An immunotherapy tablet containing grass pollen allergens is now also available in many countries. The tablet (Grazax) is dissolved under the tongue, ideally starting eight weeks before the hayfever season begins, and continued throughout the hayfever season. Grazax contains grass proteins that prime the immune system so it doesn't over-react to grass pollens.

Rescue treatment Another option for troublesome asthma symptoms consists of "rescue treatment". This involves taking corticosteroid drugs in tablet form to get your lung inflammation under control. Doctors prescribe tablets as a short course to relieve acute asthma, and you then stop taking them or tail off the dose as soon as your symptoms abate. Corticosteroid tablets quickly damp down lung inflammation: a child may need to take oral steroids for only three or four days; an adult for one or two weeks. Although oral steroids are associated with serious side effects – such as weight gain, thinning bones (osteoporosis), increased blood pressure, stretch marks, stomach ulceration, lowered immunity and reduced resistance to stress – they are unlikely to harm you when taken in short courses two or three times a year. A few people need long courses of oral steroids to control life-threatening asthma, but doctors prescribe prolonged courses only where the life-saving benefits outweigh the risks.

Please note that the inhaled steroids in your preventer medication are very different from steroid tablets and are unlikely to cause serious side effects if you use them as directed.

Personal management plans

As part of your asthma management your doctor or asthma nurse will design a treatment plan that's tailored to your symptoms and lifestyle. This will show you how to match treatment with symptoms. Sometimes you'll need to step up your asthma treatment, then, when your symptoms are under control, you can step it down again. Recognizing the early warning signs that your asthma is getting worse is critical in helping to avoid an attack. Below I give an example of a step-wise treatment program. In this example, you would return to the previous step as soon as your symptoms were controlled.

- **Step 1**: Use your reliever inhaler when you need it for symptom relief, but try to keep its use minimal. If you need to use your reliever more than twice a week, move up to step 2.
- **Step 2**: Use your preventer inhaler twice a day, plus your reliever inhaler on the occasions you need it. If this does not control your symptoms, move up to step 3.
- **Step 3**: Take a stronger dose preventer inhaler. Use your reliever inhaler as required. If your symptoms are not controlled, move up to step 4.
- **Step 4**: Use your regular preventer inhaler plus a regular protector inhaler. Use your reliever inhaler whenever you need to. If your symptoms are not controlled, move up to step 5.
- **Step 5**: Take oral steroid tablets (soluble prednisolone) in a single daily dose for four days.

Your peak flow readings

Monitoring your peak flow readings (see page 16) is an essential part of your asthma management. Keep a diary of your readings or plot them on a graph. If your peak flow readings are dropping, you can adjust your treatment in line with the advice given in your personal management plan. Ideally you will want to be in the green zone every day, because this means you are within 80–100 percent of your personal best peak flow. Make sure you know what treatment you need at times when your readings fall into the yellow or red zones – you need to take action to avoid an asthma attack. Bear in mind that when your readings fall into the red zone, this is less than 50 percent of your personal best peak flow – by this point your symptoms may be severe and you may need to go to hospital for urgent treatment.

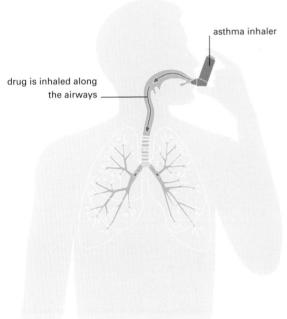

asthma inhaler

drug is inhaled along the airways

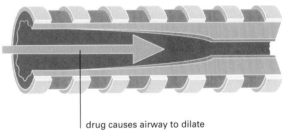

drug causes airway to dilate

Using an inhaler

Drugs to treat asthma are usually inhaled into the lungs where they act directly on the airways. When you feel breathless or wheezy, a reliever inhaler eases symptoms by relaxing the muscles in the airways, causing them to dilate. A preventer inhaler works by damping down inflammation in the lungs to stop symptoms occurring.

The natural health approach

Complementary therapies and dietary and lifestyle changes can have a profound effect on your asthma symptoms. In many cases, they work so well that you can **reduce your need for asthma medication.** In this section I describe the **complementary approaches** that are most helpful for asthma – there are quite a few of them. They include aromatherapy, herbal medicine, homeopathy, reflexology, acupuncture and acupressure, as well as movement, manipulation and relaxation therapies. Many people find that **breath control techniques,** such as the Buteyko method and yoga pranayama, have an extremely positive effect on the functioning of their lungs. **Nutritional approaches are also vitally important** – your diet can regulate the level of inflammation present in your lungs. Relatively simple steps such as cutting back on salt, and eating more fruit, vegetables, fish and certain **asthma-friendly superfoods** have the power to transform your health. I tell you how to identify your individual food intolerances and which **nutritional supplements can help to improve asthma symptoms**. I also look at the **lifestyle changes** you can make, such as avoiding your asthma triggers, managing stress, quitting smoking, losing excess weight and exercising regularly.

complementary approaches to treatment

The holistic approach to treating asthma includes a number of therapies you can use together with the medication prescribed by your doctor. In many cases, these are practitioner-led therapies – you get the most benefit from them by visiting a professional therapist for a course of treatment. However, there are also self-help techniques that you can try at home and I have included as many of these as possible on the following pages. You'll also find plenty of self-help techniques in the programs in Part Three.

The main complementary therapies that can help your asthma are aromatherapy, herbal medicine, naturopathy, homeopathy, osteopathy, chiropractic, reflexology, Rolfing, Alexander Technique, acupuncture and breath control techniques. As stress can trigger asthma, relaxation techniques such as meditation and hypnotherapy can reduce anxiety and help breathing.

When you have asthma, using complementary approaches, together with dietary and lifestyle changes, can often improve your breathing enough to reduce your need to use your reliever inhaler. It can also improve your peak flow measurements enough for you to step down your use of a preventer inhaler – always follow the instructions in the personal management plan that your doctor or asthma nurse has drawn up for you.

Consulting a therapist

When booking an appointment with a complementary practitioner, it's important to select one who is accredited with the appropriate professional organization, carries indemnity insurance and operates by an established code of conduct. Most professional organizations provide lists of registered practitioners, and many have a search facility on their website to help you locate a therapist in your area. I give the contact details of useful organizations on pages 174–175.

Having selected a qualified practitioner, ask them about their background and qualifications, and also about their specific experience and successes when treating people with asthma. It's also a good idea to find out how long your course of treatment is likely to last – and how much the therapist expects it to cost – before committing yourself to an appointment. You may find you need only one or two consultations – for example, with an homeopath or medical herbalist – to point you in the right direction. After initial guidance from a therapist you may be able to carry on treating yourself at home. With other practitioner-led therapies, such as reflexology, osteopathy and acupuncture, you may decide to attend sessions on a regular basis.

Your asthma management
Remember, if you need to use your reliever inhaler more than twice a week, you should be using your preventer inhaler every day as well. This will damp down the lung inflammation that is triggering your asthma attacks.

aromatherapy

Inhaling the scents of essential oils (derived from plants) has a healing effect on the body. Asthma is treated with inhaled drugs, so it's not surprising that inhaling some essential oils can prove beneficial for people with asthma. As well as providing symptom relief, essential oils are useful for reducing stress, and promoting relaxation and sleep.

How to use essential oils

You can inhale essential oils directly from a tissue or by diffusing them into the atmosphere using an aromatherapy water heater. You can also massage them into your skin but, because essential oils are so concentrated, you should first dilute them with a carrier oil such as avocado, almond, calendula, grapeseed, jojoba or wheatgerm oil. The exception is lavender essential oil, which you can use neat on your skin.

An oil blend should normally contain a maximum total of one drop essential oil to each 24 drops of carrier oil. This is equal to five drops of essential oil in 10ml (2 tsp) carrier oil.

Although you can use aromatherapy as a self-help technique at home, you will also gain great benefits from visiting an aromatherapist and receiving a massage with a blend of oils that have been selected specifically for you. Full treatment usually lasts 60 minutes and, at the end of a session, you will feel warm, contented and relaxed. For optimum benefit, have one or two sessions per week for a month.

Oils for treating asthma

The oils that are most beneficial for treating asthma are bergamot, camomile and lavender, and these three are commonly used in an anti-asthma blend. To make a therapeutic rub, add 1ml lavender essential oil and 5 drops of Roman camomile essential oil to 10ml

Use essential oils with caution

- Some people with asthma are sensitive to certain inhaled aromas. Avoid essential oils that seem to upset your breathing.
- Don't take essential oils internally.
- Before using an essential oil blend on your skin, put a small amount on a patch of skin and leave it for an hour to ensure you are not sensitive to it.
- Don't use essential oils if you are pregnant, or likely to be, except under specialist advice from an experienced aromatherapist.
- Keep essential oils away from your face and eyes.
- If you are taking homeopathic remedies, don't use peppermint, rosemary or lavender essential oils as these may neutralize the homeopathic effect.
- Essential oils are flammable, so don't put them on an open flame.

(2 tsp) carrier oil. Rub this into your chest at night to help you breathe while you're asleep.

For congestion that makes it difficult to breathe, inhale a few drops of eucalyptus oil on a tissue as you need to, or heat the oil in a diffuser. Alternatively, use frankincense, which promotes calm, slow, deep breathing and helps to create a meditative state.

Other useful oils are those that are anti-spasmodic (bergamot, camomile, clary-sage, lavender, marjoram, neroli and orange), anti-allergy (camomile, lavender and melissa), anti-inflammatory (bergamot, camomile, lavender and myrrh), anti-infective (bergamot, eucalyptus and lavender) and expectorant or decongestant (bergamot, eucalyptus, marjoram, myrrh, peppermint and sandalwood).

herbal medicine

Herbal medicines are made from different parts of plants, and may include extracts from the roots, flowers, leaves, bark, fruit, seeds or even stems, depending on which has the highest concentration of active components. More than a third of medically prescribed drugs are derived from traditional plant remedies, including sodium cromoglycate, an anti-asthma drug derived from the Middle Eastern herb khella. Unlike drugs, which tend to contain a single, isolated, active ingredient, herbal medicines supply a blend of natural ingredients that have a synergistic action. They therefore tend to have a more gentle action with a reduced risk of side effects (although this is not always the case).

How to use herbs

You can either visit a herbalist for professional advice or use herbalism as a self-help treatment. When buying a herbal remedy, choose a product that has been "standardized". This means it contains a known and consistent amount of active ingredients and each dose will provide the same benefits. Standardized remedies are also more likely to have clinical trials supporting their use.

Before you take a herbal remedy, check with a pharmacist or herbalist for information on possible drug–herb interactions. When starting on a herbal remedy, keep a record of your peak flow measurements at least four times a day to see what effect the herb is having on your asthma (it may take up to a month to produce the full effect). Always continue to use your prescribed asthma medication. If your peak flow measurements improve, consult your doctor about reducing your medication.

Herbs for treating asthma

You may use any of the following herbs to treat asthma. Some herbs reduce inflammation; others have an anti-spasmodic action that relaxes your airways.

Khella (*Ammi visnaga*) Khella contains a number of unique chemicals, including khellin, a powerful lung bronchodilator and anti-spasmodic, from which the cromoglycate group of anti-asthma drugs are derived. It makes your airways less likely to become inflamed in the presence of triggers such as airborne allergens. Typical dose: 600mg, once or twice a day.

Astragalus root (*Astragalus membranaceus*) Also known as huang qi or Chinese milkvetch, astragalus root is used to both treat and prevent respiratory infections. In a study of 28 people with asthma, astragalus significantly improved lung function compared with an inactive placebo.
Typical dose: 200–400mg, daily. If taken for a respiratory infection, use higher doses. Choose extracts standardized to 0.5 percent glucosides and 70 percent polysaccharides.

Frankincense (*Boswellia serrata*) This gum resin has anti-inflammatory components known as boswellic acids. Research suggests it can alleviate asthma symptoms and improve lung function.
Typical dose: 200–400mg, two or three times a day. Choose extracts standardized to contain at least 37.5 percent boswellic acids.

Coleus (*Coleus forskohlii*) Research suggests that this herb inhibits the release of histamine by the body, and relaxes the airways.
Typical dose: 50mg, once or twice a day. Select supplements standardized to contain 18 percent forskolin.

Echinacea (*Echinacea purpurea*) A potent immune-booster, echinacea is widely used to prevent and treat recurrent respiratory infections (such as the common cold), which, in turn, helps prevent secondary asthma attacks.

Typical dose: 200–300mg, three times daily as a treatment for a respiratory infection. You may take it at a low dose, long term, to prevent infections, or at a high dose when you feel an infection coming on. Follow the manufacturer's guidelines. Select products standardized to at least 3.5 percent echinicosides.

English ivy (*Hedera helix*) English ivy leaf extracts contain substances that have an anti-spasmodic action. Ivy is also used as an expectorant to thin and loosen mucus, and for its antibacterial actions. Studies suggest that ivy extracts can reduce airway resistance by at least 54 percent more than an inactive placebo.

Typical dose: 100–300mg, once or twice a day. Select products that are standardized to contain a stated amount of hederacosides.

Ginkgo biloba Ginkgo leaf extracts contain a variety of powerful antioxidants, including unique chemicals known as ginkgolides and bilobalides. These have a smooth-muscle-relaxing effect and have been shown to significantly reduce airway hyperreactivity and asthma symptoms.

Typical dose: 120mg, daily. Select extracts standardized to contain at least 24 percent ginkgolides. Don't use ginkgo leaves from garden trees; they contain chemicals that can cause allergic reactions.

Chinese basil (*Perilla frutescens*) Also known as the purple mint plant or wild coleus, this herb is used to ease spasm in the smooth muscles and to reduce allergic reactions. It can significantly improve peak flow volume and other measures of lung function after just four weeks of treatment.

Typical dose: 3g, twice a day.

Rosemary (*Rosmarinus officinalis*) Rosemary has anti-spasmodic and antioxidant actions that can ease asthma symptoms by relaxing muscles in the lungs.

Typical dose: drink an infusion three times a day (see box below).

Making a rosemary infusion

Place a handful of freshly picked rosemary leaves in a warmed glass or china teapot. Add freshly boiled water, and place the lid on the teapot. Leave to infuse for 10 minutes. Strain into a mug and drink (hot or cold), three times a day.

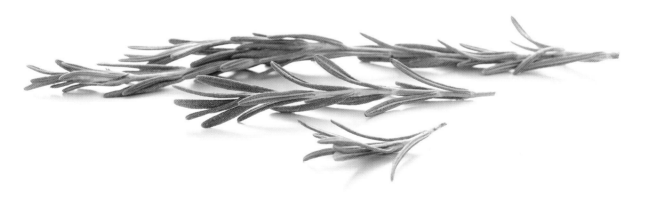

naturopathy

Naturopathy is an umbrella therapy that encompasses a range of complementary approaches. If you consult a naturopath, you'll be given advice about healthy eating, nutritional supplements, regular exercise and getting enough sleep. You may also be treated with aromatherapy, homeopathy, reflexology or acupuncture. Many naturopaths also practise iridology. This is a form of diagnosis in which health problems are recognized through changes in the eyes. Each part of your iris – the coloured part of your eye – is believed to relate to a particular area of your body, and is as unique to you as your fingerprint. Studying the iris under magnification allows the detection of inherited genetic weaknesses, along with tendencies toward certain organ or system dysfunctions.

Naturopathic treatment for asthma

Naturopaths advise following a wholefood, high-fibre – and preferably organic – diet that is low in salt, fat and additives and high in fibre and antioxidants; and that contains plenty of vegetables, nuts, seeds, wholegrains and pulses. For asthma, a naturopath will suggest that you avoid foods that promote the secretion of excess mucus. These include dairy foods and processed products made from refined white flour and/or white sugar. Instead, he or she will encourage you to eat foods that reduce mucus production, such as onions, garlic and citrus fruits; and foods that reduce inflammation, such as oily fish, and fruit and vegetables in general. A naturopath is also likely to test you for food allergies (see pages 44–45).

Some naturopaths suggest following a vegan diet if you have asthma. In one long-term study of 35 people with asthma, elimination of animal products (meaning all meat, fish, eggs and dairy products) for one year produced significant improvement in 71 percent of

people within four months, and in 92 percent after one year. Please be aware that if you follow a restricted diet such as this, it's important to take a multivitamin and mineral supplement to prevent nutritional deficiencies, especially in iron, zinc and vitamin B12.

Even if you don't follow a vegan diet, nutritional supplements are a key part of the naturopathic approach. Supplements that a naturopath will often recommend include antioxidants (such as vitamins C and E), B-group vitamins, magnesium, selenium, zinc and omega-3 fish oils. A naturopath may also use medicinal herbs (see pages 26–27) and suggest that you drink strong cocoa, coffee or tea to promote bronchodilation. This is based on the fact that cocoa contains theobromine, coffee contains caffeine and tea contains theophylline – all of which help to relax the smooth muscles of the bronchi in the lungs. Theophylline is an accepted, although now old-fashioned, medical treatment for asthma. (Avoid caffeine if you take medication containing theophylline.)

A naturopath may also treat asthma by giving you advice about relaxation and stress management. Some naturopaths apply hot compresses to your chest and back to ease lung congestion and improve your breathing. This is something you can try at home (see box, below).

A soothing chest compress
Fill a bowl with hot water and add a therapeutic essential oil blend. For example, six drops eucalyptus and six drops peppermint (see page 25). Dip a folded piece of cotton cloth, such as a teatowel or pillow case, into the scented water. Squeeze out the excess water and place the moistened cloth onto your bare chest or back until it cools to body temperature. Then repeat two or three times.

homeopathy

Homeopathy uses tiny quantities of selected substances – plants, animals or mineral deposits – to stimulate your body's healing powers. The first principle of homeopathy is that "like cures like", which is why remedies are made from substances that, at full-strength, would create the symptoms they are intended to treat. However, in tiny doses, the opposite effect occurs and symptoms improve. In the case of asthma, a homeopath may use a dilution of an agent that triggers your asthma, for example, pollen.

The second principle of homeopathy is "less cures more". Potentially noxious substances are diluted many millions of times to eradicate their undesirable side effects and enhance their healing properties. Remedies are steeped and shaken in an alcohol solution to produce a mother tincture. One drop of this mother tincture is then added to 99 drops of pure water or alcohol to produce a dilute potency known as 1c (100^{-1}). To produce a dilution with a potency of 2c, one drop of the 1c dilution is added to 99 drops of pure water or alcohol, and so on. The potency of a remedy shows how many times it has been diluted.

In one study, 28 people with allergic asthma who were sensitive to house dust mites were given either homeopathic remedies or a placebo. Within one week, those taking active remedies showed a significant reduction in their symptoms. This improvement persisted for up to eight weeks. Analysis of these results, together with those from three other trials, suggests that homeopathy is significantly more effective than a placebo at treating allergic asthma.

How to take homeopathic remedies

Take a homeopathic remedy on its own, without eating or drinking for at least 30 minutes before or afterwards. Don't handle tablets – tip them into the lid of the container or onto a spoon, then drop them in your mouth. Suck or chew them; don't swallow them whole. Other guidelines are as follows:

- Avoid drinking strong tea or coffee around the time of taking a remedy.
- Avoid using powerful essential oils such as rosemary and peppermint. ·
- If symptoms worsen initially, persevere as this is a sign that the remedy is working.
- If, after taking the remedy for the time stated, there's no obvious improvement, ask a homeopath to give you a different remedy.

Consulting a homeopath

A homeopath will assess your constitutional type, personality, lifestyle, family background, likes and dislikes, and symptoms, before selecting a remedy. Treatment often starts with a 6c or 12c potency and is taken two or three times a day. If partial relief occurs, but symptoms return once you stop taking the remedy, you may be given a 30c potency which, according to the principles of homeopathy, is more powerful.

An initial consultation with a homeopath usually lasts 45 to 60 minutes, with follow-up appointments lasting around 30 minutes. For optimum benefit, have an initial and at least one follow-up session before assessing whether or not you wish to continue. See page 175 for information on how to find a homeopath.

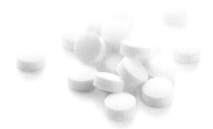

Homeopathic remedies for asthma

The following homeopathic remedies may be helpful for people with asthma. Different remedies may be recommended by a homeopath depending on your symptoms and your constitutional type.

remedy	prepared from	used to treat
Ambra grisea	Whale ambergris	Exercise-induced asthma; nervous asthma where symptoms are worse when other people are around.
Antimonium tartaricum	Antimony tartrate salt	Asthma with a rattly chest, but coughing produces little mucus.
Arsenicum album	Arsenic	Asthma that occurs soon after midnight and makes you feel anxious, restless and uncomfortable.
Kali nitricum	Potassium nitrate salt	Asthma that's accompanied by a stitch in the side of your chest.
Lachesis mutus	Bushmaster snake venom	Asthma attacks that start in the night when you are asleep, or when you wake up.
Lobelia inflata	Indian tobacco	Asthma that's preceded by prickling sensations all over your body.
Lycopodium clavatum	Club moss	Asthma that's worse in late afternoon and early evening and associated with abdominal bloating.
Naja tripudians	Cobra snake venom	Asthma accompanied by constriction in the chest and throat so you wake up gasping and choking.
Pulsatilla nigricans	Wind flower	Symptoms that are variable and come and go quickly (they tend to be worse in the evening and at night, and in hot weather).
Silicea	Silicon dioxide	Coughing that is worse on lying down and better in wet and humid conditions; asthma in people who also have sweaty feet.
Sulphur	Sulphur iodine	Symptoms that develop after a cold and in those who crave fatty food and like to keep windows open for a flow of fresh air.

osteopathy

Osteopathy was developed in the 19th century by Andrew Taylor Still, an American army doctor. The word "osteopathy" comes from the Greek *osteon*, meaning bone, and *pathos*, meaning disease. It's a method of diagnosis and treatment based on the body's musculo-skeletal system. Osteopaths believe that your muscles, ligaments, connective tissues, bones and joints don't just form a "coat-hanger" to support your body, but are also important in maintaining the health of other parts of the body such as the respiratory system. Gentle manipulation of the soft tissues and joints is used to help relax muscles, correct poor alignment, improve body function, reduce pain and restore health.

A study published in the *Journal of the American Osteopathic Association* involving 140 children with asthma found that, in those receiving osteopathic manipulation, peak flow rate increased by 25–75 percent, while those receiving simulated osteopathic manipulation showed no improvement.

Consulting an osteopath

The first time you visit an osteopath, you are asked about your general health, your current health problems and your medical history. The osteopath then performs a physical examination and assesses the range of movements in your joints. He or she uses their sense of touch to palpate (feel) parts of your body and detect any areas of weakness or excessive strain. The osteopath will check your posture for symmetry, and your pelvis for alignment, and compare the length of your legs. He or she will test your nerve reflexes by gently tapping on muscle tendons at your knee, ankle, elbows and/or wrists using a rubber reflex hammer.

Osteopaths use their hands to perform a wide range of manipulations on the body. These include gentle massage, soft tissue techniques to reduce tension, rhythmic passive joint mobilizations to improve the range of movement in a joint, and swift, high-velocity thrusts. Osteopaths are also trained in cranial osteopathy, in which the bones of the skull are gently manipulated, and/or craniosacral therapy, which involves gentle manipulation of both the skull and base of the spine. Osteopathy can help asthma in the following ways:

- Easing breathing difficulties by realigning joints.
- Easing restrictions to the chest and ribs.
- Relaxing the muscles of the respiratory system.
- Improving blood supply to the lungs.
- Improving nerve function in the lungs.

A first session with an osteopath typically lasts from 40 minutes to an hour. In addition to your treatment, you will probably be given advice on good posture when you are sitting, standing, lying down and walking. Follow-up treatments tend to last for 20–40 minutes. The average course of treatment is six to eight sessions.

Chiropractic or osteopathy?

People often wonder what the difference is between these two therapies. They actually share a common origin, and around 80 percent of the techniques used by each profession are similar, although the terminology is different. Chiropractors tend to use more diagnostic procedures such as X-rays, MRI scans, and blood and urine tests. They are more likely to push on vertebrae with their hands, whereas osteopaths use your limbs to make levered thrusts. An osteopath usually mobilizes a joint by stretching it rhythmically within its normal range.

chiropractic

Chiropractic was developed in the late 19th century by Daniel Palmer, a Canadian school teacher with an interest in anatomy and physiology. Chiropractors specialize in the diagnosis and treatment of conditions that arise from misalignments of the spinal bones (known as subluxations). Just a small movement of a vertebra away from its normal position can trap, squash or stretch a nerve, and is a common cause of pain, discomfort, reduced mobility and shallow breathing. The word "chiropractic" is derived from the Greek *cheir*, meaning "hand", and *praktikos* meaning "done-by". Chiropractors use their hands and a finely tuned sense of touch to adjust the spine and extremities where there are signs of restricted movement. The main objective is to improve aches and pains, but a chiropractor also treats disorders of the respiratory system, such as asthma.

An article published in the *Journal of Vertebral Subluxation Research* found chiropractic produced positive effects within two months in a group of children with asthma. Almost one third of the children treated with chiropractic were able to reduce their medication use as a result. In another study, chiropractic manipulation reduced the number of asthma attacks experienced by children from an average of four a month down to one – and medication use decreased by nearly 70 percent. Chiropractic can help adults, too. A study from Denmark, involving people aged between 18 and 44 with chronic asthma, compared the effects of chiropractic manipulation with placebo manipulation. Participants received treatments twice a week for four weeks. Although there were no differences between the groups in peak flow readings or daily use of inhalers, chiropractic manipulation did appear to reduce the over-sensitivity of participants' airways to various triggers. Those receiving chiropractic

manipulation also said that they felt the severity of their asthma decreased by more than a third during the course of the study.

Although not all studies show that there are benefits of chiropractic for people with asthma, it's an option that's worth exploring when other approaches haven't worked for you.

Consulting a chiropractor

During your first visit to a chiropractor, you are asked in-depth questions about your symptoms, medical history, lifestyle, diet, exercise patterns, work and the type of bed you sleep on. You may also have X-rays taken. A practitioner will observe your posture and how you walk, and will ask how you sit at a desk. During the examination you are asked to variously stand, sit or lie down on a chiropractic couch, and you are manoeuvred into a number of positions to assess your mobility, flexibility and nerve function. This "motion palpation" assessment helps the chiropractor assess which joints move freely, and which are stiff or locked.

A chiropractor uses rapid, direct, yet gentle thrusts to re-align muscles, tendons, ligaments and joints. Correcting a vertebral subluxation is called an "adjustment". Adjustments that combine a rapid thrust and immediate release help a bone move toward its correct position, often with a "click". This helps to correct poor alignment, improve mobility, relieve pain and tension, and promote relaxation. Sometimes, a rubber-tipped instrument known as an activator is used to gently manipulate the vertebrae, giving a small, precise, measured thrust. Chiropractic may also include stretching and massage techniques.

A first treatment with a chiropractor typically lasts 30 to 60 minutes, with follow-up sessions taking 15 to 20 minutes. You may need two or three treatments during the first week, followed by weekly or monthly follow-ups, although this may vary.

reflexology

Reflexology is thought to originate from India, China and Egypt, and date back more than 5,000 years. A form of reflexology, known as "zone therapy", was first practised in the West by Dr William Fitzgerald in 1913. Later on, Eunice Ingham developed Fitzgerald's work to create modern reflexology practice.

The aim of reflexology is to treat both the symptoms and the causes of illness. The therapy is based on the belief that different areas on your feet correspond to distant parts of your body, and relate to internal organs and structures and their functions. The areas – known as reflexes – on your right foot correspond to the right side of your body, and those on your left foot to the left side of your body. Similar reflexology points are also found on your hands.

Reflexology also has a diagnostic element in that, while massaging a particular zone on the foot, the therapist may identify areas of unusual tenderness or grittiness. This suggests a potential problem in the area to which that reflex relates – even if you aren't aware of any symptoms. Massaging these zones with tiny pressure movements can to help relieve or prevent problems in the corresponding part of the body.

In a study in which people with asthma received either real or simulated reflexology for 10 weeks, there were similar improvements in peak flow measurements in both groups, but a trend in favour of reflexology became significant when researchers also analyzed symptom diaries. Reflexology is certainly relaxing, which may help to reduce stress-related asthma symptoms.

Consulting a reflexologist

Reflexologists massage all areas of your feet and/or hands using firm thumb and finger pressure, and treat a specific problem such as asthma by concentrating on

Self-help reflexology

You may find it beneficial to massage the following reflexes in your foot. This takes 10 minutes. Ideally you should do it on at least two days a week (in the morning and again in the evening). You can also do it on a daily basis if you find it helpful. Use the foot maps on page 34 to help you locate the relevant reflexes.

1 Find a comfortable chair and spend a minute or two sitting quietly before you begin the massage. Bring your attention to your breathing. Don't attempt to change it in any way; just be aware of the way it flows into and out of your body. When you feel ready, bring your left foot up onto your right thigh.

2 Using your thumb, press and hold the solar plexus reflex. Then gently massage across the diaphragm line for one minute.

3 Massage along your spinal reflex, concentrating on the area at the base of your big toe to the mid-curve of your instep. Do this for one minute.

4 Massage your lung reflex, which lies between the diaphragm line and the base of your toes. Do this for one minute.

5 Massage the bronchial tube reflex, which runs between the inner end of the diaphragm line up to between your first and second toes. Do this for one minute.

6 Finally, massage inside the arch of your foot, which contains a reflex relating to your adrenal gland. Do this for one minute.

7 Repeat the massage on your right foot.

the relevant reflexes. These usually include the solar plexus, spine (emphasizing the thoracic vertebrae), the diaphragm line, the bronchial tube and the lung reflexes. Stimulating these areas relieves upper-body tension and inflammation, and improves breathing.

The lung reflexes are located on the balls of both feet, above your diaphragm line (see illustration), while the solar plexus area is just below the diaphragm line on the left foot. The spine reflex runs along the inner edges of your feet, with the thoracic vertebrae in the area between the base of your big toe to the mid-curve of your instep. Your bronchial tube reflex runs from between the first (big) and second toes and curves down to the inner edge of the diaphragm line.

Reflexology treatment usually lasts 45 to 60 minutes and, at the end of each session, you will usually feel warm, contented and relaxed. For optimum benefits, have one session per week for two months, then assess whether or not you wish to continue. To find a therapist go to page 175.

Reflexes on the soles of the feet
These reflexology "foot maps" show some of the reflexes that correspond with major body organs. If you have asthma, a reflexologist is likely to work on your lung, solar plexus and spine reflexes, among others.

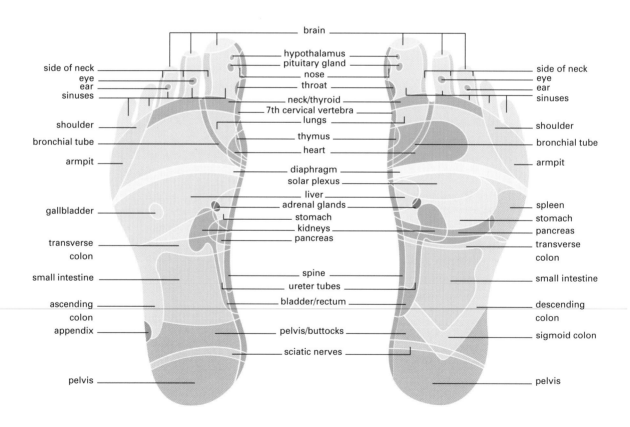

side of neck · eye · ear · sinuses · shoulder · bronchial tube · armpit · gallbladder · transverse colon · small intestine · ascending colon · appendix · pelvis

brain · hypothalamus · pituitary gland · nose · throat · neck/thyroid · 7th cervical vertebra · lungs · thymus · heart · diaphragm · solar plexus · liver · adrenal glands · stomach · kidneys · pancreas · spine · ureter tubes · bladder/rectum · pelvis/buttocks · sciatic nerves

side of neck · eye · ear · sinuses · shoulder · bronchial tube · armpit · spleen · stomach · pancreas · transverse colon · small intestine · descending colon · sigmoid colon · pelvis

rolfing and alexander technique

Rolfing

Developed in the 1940s by Dr Ida Rolf, an American biochemist, Rolfing is designed to correct distortions of the body caused by the effects of gravity, and physical or emotional trauma. The body is viewed like a stack of bricks, which are stressed and misaligned owing to poor posture. However, when the body regains its correct posture, the stack becomes stable again.

Anecdotal reports suggest that Rolfing can improve breathing in people with asthma, but there has been no research to confirm its effectiveness.

Consulting a therapist During a session you lie down and are guided through a series of movements, to which you are asked to synchronize your breathing. The therapist slowly stretches and repositions your body's supportive soft tissues, rather like a sculptor, to correct misalignments, free restrictions, reduce tension and pain, and improve well-being. A fundamental aim of Rolfing is to maximize the capacity of the ribcage to allow the lungs to expand to their fullest, so that breathing is optimally efficient.

Treatment usually consists of 10 sessions of one hour each. The therapist massages your tissues using his or her hands and elbows. He or she may apply their body weight during deep tissue work.

Alexander Technique (AT)

Australian actor Frederick Alexander developed the Alexander Technique in the 1930s based on the belief that poor posture and faulty body movements contribute to illnesses such as asthma. Alexander's theory was that, over time, persistent bad postural habits such as hunching your shoulders, slouching, and tensing up owing to anxiety affects the spine and nervous system, which, in turn, affects the function of your internal organs, such as your lungs in the case of asthma. Studies published 20 to 30 years ago show that AT can improve breathing, but no recent research has been carried out.

Consulting a therapist AT is usually taught on a one-to-one basis. You are taught to recognize "patterns of misuse" in your everyday movements. You pay attention to the way you stand, and the alignment of your head, neck and spine, so you begin to move in a more balanced, relaxed and fluid way. Gentle exercises and movements teach you how to move correctly so your chest can expand fully and your breathing can improve. To learn AT, you will usually need between 15 and 30 lessons, held twice weekly, each lasting between 30 and 45 minutes.

What is Hellerwork?

A modern adaptation of Rolfing, Hellerwork combines massage and postural adjustments with movement re-education exercises to rebalance the link between mind and body. Hellerwork was devised in the late 1970s by Joseph Heller, an American engineer who applied the mechanical principles he had learned to the human body in order to improve health and vitality. Massage under the ribcage helps to release tension within the diaphragm and makes breathing easier. As well as using deep pressure and manipulation techniques, Hellerwork also involves the exploration of emotions triggered by the release of tension.

acupuncture

Acupuncture is a technique from Traditional Chinese Medicine. It's based on the principle that life-force energy, called qi or chi, needs to flow freely through the body to ensure good health. Qi flows through channels called meridians and becomes concentrated at certain points (called acupoints) where it can enter or leave the body. Acupuncture needles are inserted into these acupoints where they have a therapeutic effect on the flow of qi.

Factors such as stress, poor diet and spiritual neglect can easily disrupt the flow of qi through the meridians. A disrupted or imbalanced flow of qi is believed to be responsible for the symptoms of illness. In Traditional Chinese Medicine, asthma is believed to result from energy blockages along a number of different meridians, including the lung meridian, as well as the stomach and kidney meridians where they cross the chest. Several points on the bladder meridian, where it crosses the upper back, are also used to treat asthma – the severity of asthma symptoms is thought to increase as a result of blocked qi in the back.

In a recent study of children aged between six and 12 years, published in the journal of the European Society of Pediatric Allergy and Immunology, the combination of laser acupuncture (see below) plus probiotics (see page 61) improved peak flow by 17 percent compared with only two percent in those receiving sham treatment. Studies of adults with asthma have also shown that acupuncture used in conjunction with medical treatments can improve symptoms and general well-being, with some people experiencing immediate widening of the airways after acupuncture, and a 20 percent improvement in the amount of air they could breathe out in one second. Not all studies have found acupuncture to be beneficial. However, the studies that haven't revealed

Self-help acupressure

Stimulate these acupoints to relieve asthma. Work on each point initially, then just the one/s you find most helpful. Do this twice a day, morning and evening, on two or three days a week (or every day if you wish).

- Stomach 16 – this is on the front of your chest on each side, just below your third rib, and directly above your nipple. Press lightly, then increase the pressure. Release gradually then build up pressure again – hold for one minute.
- Lung 1 – touch the ends of your collarbones (clavicles) and move your hands slowly downward until your middle fingers find a tender, knotted spot on each side. Breathe in and press firmly for a few seconds. Breathe out and repeat.
- Urinary bladder 13 (see also page 150) – reach over your left shoulder with your right hand to between your shoulder blade and spine, one finger-width below the level of the upper tip of your shoulder blade. Press firmly, take five long deep breaths then release. Repeat on your right shoulder.

a therapeutic effect tend to be those that look at a one-size-fits-all approach to asthma (as opposed to acupuncture treatment that's tailored to the individual).

Consulting an acupuncturist

Before you receive treatment an acupuncturist will ask you detailed questions about your current health, lifestyle and diet. During your treatment sterile, disposable, acupuncture needles will be inserted a few millimetres into your skin at key acupoints. You may notice a slight pricking, tingling or buzzing as the needle is inserted or rotated but you shouldn't feel any unpleasant discomfort. Needles are usually left in place for 10 to 30 minutes and flicked or rotated to stimulate

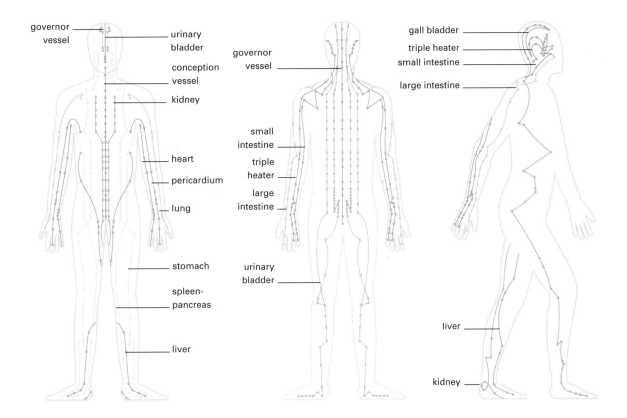

qi and to draw or disperse energy from the point. In some cases, needles are stimulated with electricity (electroacupuncture) or by burning a small cone of a dried Chinese herb (moxa) near the point. The latter is known as moxibustion. Acupoints can also be stimulated with a pen that emits laser light – children tend to find this more acceptable than needles.

An initial consultation usually lasts 45 to 60 minutes, with follow-up appointments lasting around 30 minutes. For a complex, long-standing problem such as asthma, you will benefit from having one or two treatments per week for at least two months. I've included information on how to find a practitioner at the end the book.

The meridians

There are 12 pairs of meridians in the body. To treat asthma, an acupuncturist is likely to treat specific acupoints along the lung, stomach, kidney and bladder meridians. He or she may do this with needles or a laser pen (the latter is most commonly used on children).

Acupressure

Stimulating acupoints using finger pressure is an alternative that many people find more acceptable than the insertion of needles. It's also a convenient self-help technique. I describe the three main acupressure points for asthma in the box on the opposite page.

breath control techniques

People tend to take breathing for granted because, except during an asthma attack, it happens with little effort or thought. However, the way you breathe habitually can have an impact on your asthma. In particular, overbreathing (taking in more air than you need) can lead to breathlessness and muscle spasms. Learning to breathe properly can reduce the incidence and severity of attacks. And, when you do have an attack, breathing exercises can help to calm you.

The Buteyko method

Developed by a Russian doctor, Professor Konstantin Buteyko, in the 1950s, the Buteyko method involves breathing exercises and relaxation techniques. Buteyko suggested that overbreathing leads to respiratory problems such as asthma, because it causes you to lose excess amounts of carbon dioxide, the waste acidic gas produced by cells. As a result, your blood loses acidity and becomes too alkaline. Your airways respond to this by constricting to help prevent further loss of carbon dioxide. The net result is that you struggle to breathe.

Buteyko's theory is supported by the recent finding that people with asthma have significantly lower resting levels of carbon dioxide than normal. Research shows that low levels of carbon dioxide can trigger the smooth muscles of the airways to constrict, while raised levels of carbon dioxide make them dilate. This seems to apply only to people with asthma though.

Buteyko believed that teaching people with asthma to underbreathe could raise their carbon dioxide levels and dilate their airways without medication. One study involving 600 adults with asthma found that, after six months, the Buteyko method relieved asthma symptoms by 98 percent and reduced the use of reliever medication by 98 percent (and preventer medication by 92 percent). These improvements persisted after 12 months. Those not using the method showed no significant improvements.

Buteyko breathing exercises These involve a controlled reduction in breathing, known as slow breathing and reduced breathing, together with breath-holding techniques, such as the control pause and extended pause. Buteyko also promotes the benefits of nasal breathing over mouth breathing. The latter cools and dries your airways, which can make them irritable and sensitive. In contrast, nasal breathing warms, filters and humidifies air. One study found that decreasing nocturnal mouth breathing halved night-time asthma.

Here's a simple Buteyko exercise that helps to increase your carbon dioxide level: breathe in normally then let out a little bit of air so your lungs are not full. Pinch your nose closed and hold your breath, with your mouth closed, for five seconds after you first experience the desire to breathe in (don't be tempted to hold your breath for as long as you can). When you start breathing again, breathe in and out as little as possible. See Part Three for more Buteyko exercises.

The part of the Buteyko theory that is most controversial is the concept that asthma inhalers make the problem worse by stopping your natural "breathe less" response. My advice is: by all means practise Buteyko breathing exercises, but continue to use your inhalers exactly as prescribed by your doctor, stepping down their use only as your symptoms improve.

Yogic breath control

The ancient Indian art of yogic breath control is known as pranayama. Research shows that pranayama exercises can reduce lung reactivity in people with asthma (meaning that more of a trigger is required to cause an asthma attack).

Pranayama exercises There are a variety of yogic breathing exercises in Part Three for you to try. Here's a good one to start with: Viloma Pranayama Stage I. It involves "interrupted breathing" and has a lot in common with the Buteyko method. Do it once a day.

- Lie down quietly with your eyes closed.
- Breathe in for two or three seconds and pause, holding your breath for two or three seconds.
- Continue to breathe in for another two or three seconds before pausing again. Repeat until your lungs are full (normally four or five pauses).
- Breathe out slowly and steadily. Empty your lungs.
- Breathe normally before repeating the interrupted inhalation once more.

Do you overbreathe?
Even if you breathe three or four times the volume of air you actually need, you may feel as if you are breathing normally (this is referred to as "hidden hyperventilation"). Ask a friend to count your breathing rate when you're not aware they're doing it. The average breathing rate is 10 to 12 breaths per minute, but people who overbreathe take 15 to 20 breaths per minute, and someone who is in a state of panic may take as many as 30 breaths per minute.

Exhaling too much carbon dioxide
According to Buteyko theory, overbreathing leads to excess carbon dioxide passing out of the blood and back into the alveoli, from where it is exhaled. This triggers a chain of events that results in narrowing of the airways.

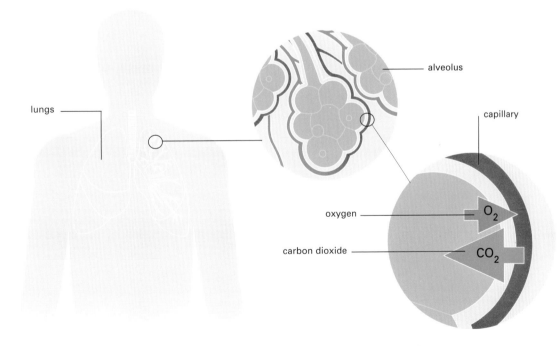

lungs

alveolus

capillary

oxygen — O_2

carbon dioxide — CO_2

relaxation therapies

When you are relaxed, your breathing is slower, and levels of the stress hormones that can trigger spasms of the airways are also reduced. I suggest that you try to fit relaxation techniques into your daily life – a number of different methods are available, and I introduce some of them here. You'll also find relaxation techniques in the programs in Part Three.

Autogenic training

Developed in 1932 by German psychiatrist Johannes Schultz, autogenic training involves a series of simple visualization exercises and verbal cues that are designed to reduce stress and promote profound relaxation. Exercises include statements such as: "My breathing is calm and regular" and are best learned by watching an instructor. They are usually performed for 15 minutes, three times a day. Autogenic training can help you breathe more slowly to combat hyperventilation and asthma symptoms. In a trial involving 41 people with asthma, autogenic training produced significant improvements in lung function.

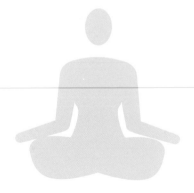

Meditation

Meditation involves concentrating your awareness on the present moment – this stills your mind and puts you in a state of relaxed alertness. When you are experienced in meditation, you can quickly enter a trance-like state in which your brain generates special theta waves that are associated with creativity, visions and profound relaxation. People who meditate regularly have higher levels of melatonin – nature's sleep-enhancing hormone – and enjoy improved sleep quality and reduced pain perception. They also have significantly better respiratory function and less need for asthma inhalers.

There is a wide variety of techniques you can use to get into a meditative state. You can focus on an image, such as a mandala; on a colour; on the rhythm of your breath; on a sound, such as "om"; on a word or phrase with personal meaning, such as "relax"; or on a physical object, such as a candle flame. Some methods of meditation, such as t'ai chi, involve movement; others, such as yoga, involve holding a particular pose in which the spine is kept straight (for example, the lotus position). Even playing with objects such as pebbles or worry beads in a rhythmic, repetitive manner can still your mind.

One study of 21 people found their asthma significantly improved while practising meditation for three months, compared with a three-month period in which they did not meditate.

If you haven't meditated before, start with 15 to 20 minutes a day, then increase this by about five minutes a week, until you get to 30 minutes a day. You'll find it beneficial to meditate five days a week, and preferably every day. Start with the technique in the box opposite.

Massage

Therapeutic touch in the form of massage has always been one of the most powerful ways to relax the body and calm the mind. Massage stimulates the release of the body's endorphins (which relieve pain and bring about feelings of well-being), eases muscle tension and stress, and promotes relaxation. In a study of 19 people with asthma, receiving a 15-minute upper-body massage once a week for 12 weeks decreased chest tightness, wheeziness and fatigue.

During massage, the soft tissues of the body are stimulated with a variety of strokes: rubbing, drumming, kneading, wringing, friction and deep pressure. Depending on the training of the therapist, massage may include the stimulation of acupoints to balance the flow of qi energy throughout your body (see page 36), or the therapist may rub diluted essential oils with anti-spasmodic or decongestant properties (see page 25) into your skin.

Visualization

This is a technique in which the powers of imagination, auto-suggestion and positive thought are used to promote relaxation. Visualization literally helps you picture your way out of a stressful situation to achieve calmness and an uplifted mood. Guided visualization involves listening to a therapist or relaxation tape to focus your breathing and conjure up a pleasant, relaxing image, such as a sun-drenched tropical beach. To help deal with a particular health problem such as asthma, you are encouraged to picture an image in your mind that represents a symptom, and then to imagine it away.

Mindful breathing
Sit comfortably and close your eyes. Take a few long, slow breaths. As you breathe out, step back from your thoughts and everything that is happening in your life. Instead bring your awareness to the present moment by focusing exclusively on your breath. Breathe normally but "watch" each breath as it flows into and out of you. (Think of this as an observation exercise rather than a breathing exercise.) Find a place within your body where you feel the sensation of breathing most clearly – let your attention rest here. If you notice your mind wandering, gently bring it back to observe the sensations of breathing. When you feel ready, slowly open your eyes, stretch and enjoy the sense of calm energy that flows through you.

Quick calming visualization

Sit comfortably with your eyes closed. Picture your airways as the branches of an upside-down tree.

Imagine warm, pine-scented air flowing along the branches. Allow your airways to expand so they can fill with fragrant air.

Do this for a few minutes, several times a day, or whenever you want to relax or breathe more easily.

nutritional approaches to treatment

There is good evidence that the increasing incidence of allergies such as asthma is linked to our diet. The most important nutritional advice I can give you – apart from avoiding foods that trigger your asthma – is to improve the balance of fats in your diet. Our ancestors evolved on a Stone Age, hunter-gatherer diet of green plants, wild animals and fish, which contained equal amounts of omega-6 fatty acids (from natural vegetable oils) and omega-3 fatty acids (from oily fish). Our diet has changed enormously since the Stone Age and we now eat up to 12 times more omega-6s than omega-3s. Researchers believe this is a key cause of inflammatory conditions such as asthma. On the opposite page I also describe some other important dietary measures you can take.

Cut down on omega-6s You don't need to cut out omega-6s altogether, as both omega-6s and omega-3s have important functions in the body (for example, GLA, an omega-6 fatty acid in evening primrose oil, is important for hormone balance, skin health and protecting against depression). You just

need to balance your intake more appropriately (see box opposite). You can cut out excess omega-6s by consuming less:

- Vegetable oil (except olive, flax seed/linseed, walnut, almond, macadamia, avocado, hempseed and rapeseed oils, which contain omega-3s and/or monounsaturated fats).
- Meat.
- Margarine.
- Fast-food and processed or manufactured foods, such as biscuits, cakes, sweets and pastries.

Eat more omega-3s Eat oily fish, such as herring, mackerel, sardine, tuna and salmon regularly (see page 58). Also eat more nuts, such as walnuts, almonds and macadamias; and take omega-3 supplements (see page 61).

Concentrate on eating fruit and vegetables
Researchers have found that people with a high intake of fruit and vegetables have better lung function and

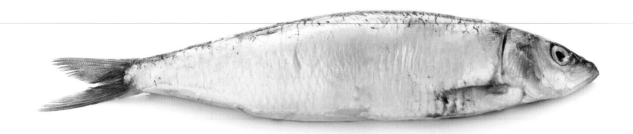

Getting the omega balance right
Omega-6s and omega-3s belong to a group of fats known as polyunsaturated fatty acids (PUFAs). Your body processes omega-6s in a different way from omega-3s, with the result that the former promote inflammation in the body and the latter fight inflammation. To discourage inflammation in the body (including the lungs), your diet needs to contain no more than three times the amount of omega-6s than omega-3s (a typical Western diet contains between seven and 12 times more). In practical terms, this means cutting down on omega-6s and eating more omega-3s.

are less likely to develop asthma – this effect is even stronger among smokers, whose need for antioxidants is greater. Children who eat the least amount of vegetables are most likely to wheeze. Dark green leafy vegetables are particularly beneficial. I recommend a diet providing plenty of raw fruit and vegetables for their vitamin, mineral, antioxidant and fibre content.

Reduce your meat consumption Meats contain a variety of "foreign" proteins that are potential allergens. It's also possible that eating meat increases the production of substances called leukotrienes, which contribute to inflammatory reactions such as asthma. If you're used to eating meat once a day or more, I suggest you cut back to eating meat three times a week or less to see if this helps your symptoms.

Lower your salt intake High-salt diets have been linked with asthma in some studies but not in others. Salt encourages fluid retention and is thought to increase lung congestion and make airways more likely to constrict. As salt is linked with other health problems such as high blood pressure, kidney

problems and coronary heart disease, it . to cut back on it anyway.

Drink enough fluid Ensure you drink enough fluid to help liquefy mucus. Aim to drink up to three litres (106fl oz) a day; more if it's hot or you exercise a lot.

Pinpoint food intolerances Identify and avoid foods that trigger your asthma, such as cow's milk, eggs, peanuts, wheat, citrus fruits and food additives. I discuss food intolerances over the next few pages.

Eat superfoods As well as fruit and vegetables and foods that are rich in omega-3 fatty acids, a number of other foods are beneficial for people with asthma. These include garlic, coffee, green tea, yogurt, ginger, turmeric, mustard and camomile (see pages 56–59).

Take appropriate supplements People with asthma can benefit from taking selected nutritional supplements, which have a powerful protective effect on your respiratory system (see pages 60–61).

Take digestive enzymes Normally, around 15 percent of the general population have low levels of hydrochloric acid in their stomach, a problem known as hypochlorhydria. Back in the 1930s, researchers discovered this was much more common in people – particularly women – with asthma, affecting between 40 and 60 percent of adults and 80 percent of children with asthma. People with asthma also appear to secrete too few digestive enzymes, especially those made in the pancreas. We don't yet fully understand why this is the case, but researchers have found that there is a definite relationship between the severity of hypochlorhydria and the severity of asthma, and taking supplements that contain weak digestive acids and enzymes can help. See page 61 for more details.

identifying food intolerances

Asthma attacks may be linked to an intolerance to a particular food or foods. There are several ways to discover if this is the case. Traditionally, people have used the elimination diet, but this is time consuming and the guidelines can be difficult to follow precisely. As a result, a number of other tests have been developed to help identify foods to which you are intolerant. Most of these are available only privately. While some tests may be useful, many are controversial or have little evidence to support them.

Elimination diets

The traditional approach to identifying foods that trigger mild to moderate asthma is an elimination and challenge diet. The simplest version of this involves removing suspect foods from your diet, then sequentially re-introducing them to see which, if any, provoke your asthma symptoms. (You choose your suspect foods by keeping a food-and-symptom diary for at least one week.) You should test foods that you suspect may cause severe asthma reactions only under medical supervision, and only if absolutely necessary to confirm the diagnosis.

A more advanced type of elimination diet involves following a bland, hypoallergenic diet that initially allows you to eat only a few limited items, typically:

- Grains: white rice or tapioca.
- Fruit: pears, pear juice and cranberries.
- Vegetables: squash, carrots, parsnips, lettuce, lentils and split peas.
- Meat: lamb, wild game and turkey.

When first starting an elimination diet, symptoms often worsen on days two to four, improve by days five to seven and disappear by days 10 to 14. When you are symptom-free you start to re-introduce eliminated foods one by one, usually at three-day intervals, while keeping a detailed food-and-symptom diary to identify problem foods. If an adverse reaction occurs, you continue to avoid the test food and wait 48 hours after all symptoms have improved before testing another.

IgG blood tests

Measuring the blood levels of an antibody known as IgG may reveal a food intolerance. The test involves collecting a small pin-prick of blood that you send off to a lab. Test kits to take the sample are available from many pharmacies. The blood is subjected to sophisticated testing that identifies the presence of raised levels of IgG against more than 100 food antigens. Avoiding foods to which you have a raised IgG level may help relieve asthma, but there haven't yet been any clinical trials to confirm this.

White blood cell analysis

White blood cells defend your body against substances that are foreign, or perceived as foreign, including some foods. Laboratory observation of the reaction

Hair mineral analysis

Although hair mineral analysis may sometimes be presented as a test for food allergies, it is not capable of identifying them. Hair mineral analysis can assess low or raised levels of minerals and trace elements in the body, but, despite the fact that a lack of some minerals (for example, magnesium and selenium; see page 60) is associated with asthma, no conclusions can be reached about your sensitivity to specific foods.

of white blood cells to more than 100 different foods, may reveal those foods to which you are sensitive.

Foods to which your white blood cells don't respond are printed in a green list meaning that you can eat them freely. Foods to which your white blood cells show varying reactions (from "bristling" to the release of all their immune chemicals and cell death) are included on an "avoid" list. You are advised to eat only foods from your green list for at least five weeks. You then re-introduce some of your "avoid" foods, starting with those that produced the mildest cell reactions. There haven't yet been any clinical trials to confirm the efficacy of white blood cell analysis.

Vega testing

Vega testing is a technique that has its roots in acupuncture and homeopathy. Its underlying principle is that we can measure abnormal bodily responses via changes in the skin's conductivity. The original VEGA electrodermal test measures electromagnetic conductivity in the body using a device known as a Wheatstone bridge galvanometer. One electrode is placed over an acupuncture point and the other is held in your hand. A glass vial containing a homeopathic dilution of the test food is then placed within the circuit – if this produces a fall in electromagnetic conductivity, it's said to indicate an allergy or intolerance to that test food. New computerized versions of the original VEGA system test for 3,500 allergens in three minutes. VEGA testing is controversial as results are inconsistent.

Applied kinesiology

This is a complementary therapy that diagnoses food allergies by assessing the strength and tone of certain muscles. A practitioner gently places light pressure on your arm to see how much resistance the muscle gives while you hold a food allergen in a glass vial in your

Intolerances versus allergies

Your asthma may be linked to either a food allergy or a food intolerance. Allergies, such as a peanut allergy, produce acute symptoms rapidly – sometimes within seconds – and, in severe cases, can be life-threatening. Intolerances, on the other hand, produce symptoms much more slowly, and are not directly life-threatening. Food allergies are easier to diagnose than intolerances – a blood test can measure the levels of a specific antibody (IgE antibody) that the body produces during an allergic reaction.

other hand. If the muscle power in your arm decreases, the test is positive for an intolerance to the food you're holding. Research comparing the results of this method with established laboratory tests for food intolerance in children and adolescents with asthma has produced inconsistent results.

Provocation-neutralization

Provocation-neutralization therapy has elements in common with immunotherapy (see page 20), but it uses more dilute solutions of allergen. Injections are given at 10-minute intervals using progressively weaker extracts of a suspected food allergen. A therapist assesses the size of the wheal that occurs around the injection site, along with your response. If the wheal gets bigger, or symptoms appear, the therapist identifies a food allergy. The first dilution that doesn't cause an increase in wheal size after 10 minutes, and/or relieves your symptoms, is called the neutralization or treatment dose. Neutralization doses of different allergens are combined and used as a treatment "vaccine". Studies of the efficacy of this therapy have produced inconsistent results.

eliminating sulfites

As many as one in 10 people with asthma have a sulfite hypersensitivity that can trigger an attack. The people most at risk are those with chronic asthma; those dependent on steroid treatments; and those who are sensitive to aspirin. Following a sulfite elimination diet such as the one in the moderate program (see pages 110–141) will help you to identify whether you have a sulfite sensitivity. If you do, you're likely to get classic asthma symptoms when you consume food or drinks containing sulfites, or when you inhale sulfite fumes (for example, when opening a bag of dried apricots). Sulfite sensitivity can also cause flushing; skin irritation or a rash; abdominal pain; diarrhea; nausea or vomiting; dizziness and faintness; swelling of the mouth and face; and difficulty swallowing. In rare cases, loss of consciousness can occur.

What are sulfites?

Sulfites (also spelled sulphites) are a group of antioxidant preservatives used in foods, drinks and some medications. They are used to preserve colour; to slow the browning of fruit, vegetables and seafood; to bleach food starches; and to condition bread dough.

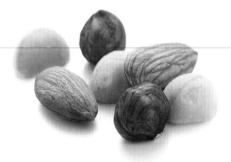

Sulfites in medications
If you have a sulfite sensitivity, it's important to avoid foods that contain high levels of sulfites, but you should also avoid drugs containing sulfites, such as some eye drops and injectable medications. The exception to this is injectable adrenaline (epinephrine). Although it contains a small amount of sulfite to prevent oxidation and inactivation of the drug, it can be life-saving for people experiencing a severe allergic reaction. So its beneficial effects far outweigh the possible adverse effects from the small amount of sulfite it contains. (Sulfites are also used to sterilize some food-grade plastic bags – you may experience a reaction when handling them.)

For example, dried apricots stay bright orange when sulfites are added, but go dull and brown without them.

At one time, sulfites were added to most fresh fruit and vegetables, especially lettuce, but, as a result of an increase in sensitivity reactions, they are now used only where no suitable alternative exists.

Food labels in many countries, such as the UK, must declare sulfiting agents where their concentration is more than 10 parts per million (ppm) or more than 10mg per kilogram or per litre – concentrations below this do not usually cause problems except in people with severe hypersensitivity. When checking food labels for the presence of sulfites, look for any of the following: sulfur dioxide, sodium sulfite,

Nuts – a good source of molybendum
Sulfite sensitivity may be linked to a deficiency of molybendum, a trace element that is found in nuts, among other foods.

Foods containing sulfites

Sulfites are added to a wide range of dried, frozen and processed foods. They bind strongly to proteins, starches and sugars in foods, which means that you can't wash them off – even with detergent – and they're not broken down during cooking. Sulfites also occur naturally in some foods, including all fermented beverages and wines (so organic wines are not necessarily sulfite-free). This table shows foods that may contain sulfites (although not all food manufacturers use them).

potential level	concentration	food
very high	greater than 100 ppm sulfites	bamboo shoots, coconut (desiccated), coleslaw (commercial), dehydrated fruits and vegetables, dried fruits and vegetables, fruit juices, ginger (dried or preserved), grapes and grape juice, lemon juice (bottled), lime juice (bottled), molasses, pickled vegetables such as pickled onions or pickled red cabbage, potatoes (frozen, processed or instant), preserved cut fruit, vegetable salads, sauerkraut, sundried tomatoes, tomato pastes (and ketchup and purée), trail mix
high	50–100 ppm sulfites	citrus peel, dried potatoes, fruit fillings and toppings, glacé fruits, maraschino cherries, sauces (such as mint sauce/jelly), wine vinegars
moderately high	10–49 ppm sulfites	breakfast cereals containing dried fruit and/or coconut (for example, muesli or granola), burgers, cheese, cider, cider vinegar, clams (tinned or bottled), corn starch, corn syrup, dextrose, fruit juices and soft drinks, gelatine, glucose syrup, gravy, guacamole, jams and jellies (not all), maple syrup, mincemeat, mushrooms (sliced and frozen), pectin, pickles and relishes, pastry shells (frozen), pizza dough (frozen), pork pies and other preserved meats, potato crisps, sausages, seafood (processed shrimp, prawns, crab, lobster, crayfish, and squid, for example, in seafood soup), tuna (canned)

sodium bisulfite, sodium hydrogen sulfite, sodium metabisulfite, potassium metabisulfite, potassium sulfite, calcium sulfite, calcium hydrogen sulfite and potassium hydrogen sulfite. Sodium dithionite can also act as a sulfiting agent.

If you see "sulfates" or "sulphates" on a food label, don't worry – these have a different chemical structure to sulfites and aren't associated with sensitivities.

How do sulfites cause symptoms?

There are several ways in which sulfites are thought to cause problems in people with asthma. The most likely explanation is that, when sulfites dissolve in the mouth during chewing, tiny amounts of sulfuric acid are formed, which releases sulfur dioxide gas. When inhaled into the lungs, this noxious gas acts as a direct irritant to hypersensitive airways to cause spasm.

reducing salicylates

Aspirin (acetylsalicylic acid) is a salicylate drug that has been used for more than 110 years to treat pain and reduce fever. One in five adults with asthma have a sensitivity to aspirin, which can trigger an attack. For this reason, people with a salicylate sensitivity must avoid all aspirin-containing painkillers and some related non-steroidal anti-inflammatory drugs (NSAIDs), such as ibuprofen. Similar substances to aspirin are present in many foods; for example, fruit, vegetables, nuts, seeds, herbs and spices. Although it's not proven that food salicylates trigger asthma, it's worth trying a low-salicylate diet such as the one in the full-strength program (see pages 142–173) to see if this helps your asthma when no other dietary approach has worked.

Salicylate sensitivity is rare in children. It tends to affect adults aged between 20 and 40, or older, and is associated with nasal inflammation (rhinitis), sinusitis, recurrent nasal polyps and a loss of sense of smell (anosmia). Exposure to salicylates may lead to skin rashes, facial swelling, lung inflammation, airway spasm and wheezing and, in extreme cases, collapse and death (this is very rare).

Doctors may diagnose salicylate sensitivity by giving you aspirin under close medical supervision – however, this is potentially dangerous. Following the full-strength program is a gentler way to find out whether or not you are sensitive to salicylates in food.

What are salicylates?

Aspirin is a synthetic salicylate originally developed after investigation of traditional herbal painkillers, such as willow bark and meadowsweet, which contain natural salicylic acid. We now know that many plants produce salicylic acid, which acts as a defence against infection. Some researchers have suggested that the high concentration of salicylic acid in fruits and vegetables may explain why vegetarians tend to experience less heart disease and bowel cancer than meat eaters.

How do salicylates cause symptoms?

Salicylates block the action of an enzyme called COX-1, the result of which is thought to be an increased production of leukotrienes. These are powerful inflammatory chemicals that cause inflammation in the nose, sinuses and lungs. The reason why some people but not others get symptoms is unclear. One theory is that people with salicylate sensitivity may have abnormal leukotriene receptors.

Tartrazine (see page 50–51) can also increase the production of leukotrienes. Up to one in four people with salicylate-exacerbated asthma are also sensitive to tartrazine. Some are also sensitive to sulfites.

Salicylates in non-food products

If you have a salicylate sensitivity, you should avoid drugs containing salicylates. Check medication labels and avoid those containing: acetylsalicylate, acetylsalicylic acid, aspirin, phenyl salicylates, salicylic acid, salicylate and salicylamide. This is not a complete list, so always check with your pharmacist or doctor. Some topical products also contain salicylates that may be absorbed through the skin. If you have a severe salicylate sensitivity, check the ingredient lists on all topical products, especially: acne cleansers and creams, arthritis pain-relieving rubs, astringents, anti-dandruff shampoos, exfoliating moisturizers, facial masks and scrubs, muscle and sports pain-relieving creams, high-strength sunblock, wart treatments and wintergreen-scented oils.

Foods containing salicylates

Most of us consume between 10 and 200mg salicylates per day in our food. The following chart shows the common dietary sources of salicylates. For more information on reducing salicylates, see the full-strength program (pages 142–173).

potential level	salicylate concentration	food
exceptionally high	greater than 4mg/100g (but spices are often eaten in tiny amounts)	asparagus, aniseed, cardamom, cayenne, celery seed, cinnamon, cloves, cumin, currants, curry powder, dates, dill, fenugreek, gherkins, ginger, licorice, mace, marjoram, mint, mustard seed, oregano, paprika, pepper (black), prunes, raisins, raspberries, rosemary, sage, stock cubes, tarragon, thyme, turmeric, Worcestershire sauce, yeast extracts
very high	2–4mg/100g	almonds, apricots, basil, commercial tomato sauces, honey, oranges, pineapple, tea leaves
high	1–2mg/100g	cantaloupe melon, Champagne, chicory, coffee, cranberries, grapes, green peppers, green olives, endive, courgettes, peanuts, pepper (white), radishes, strawberries, vanilla essence
moderate	0.5–1mg/100g	aubergine, avocado, broad beans, broccoli, cherries, chillies, cucumber, Granny Smith apples, grapefruit, grape juice, macadamias, okra, peach, pine nuts, pistachios, potatoes (especially the skins), squash, spinach (fresh), watercress, wine
low	0.1–0.5mg/100g	apple (Jonathan, Red Delicious, Golden Delicious), brandy, brazil nuts, Brussels sprouts, carrots, cashews, cauliflower, cider, coconut (desiccated), coriander leaves, corn-on-the-cob, figs (fresh), garden peas, garlic, grapefruit juice, green beans, hazelnuts, kiwi fruit, leeks, lemon, lentils, lychees (canned), mangoes, mushrooms, onions, papaya, parsley, parsnips, passion fruit, peanut butter, pear (Williams), pecans, pineapple juice, plums, pomegranate, pumpkin, red cabbage, rhubarb, rosehip tea, sesame seeds, spinach (frozen), sweet potatoes, sunflower seeds, tomatoes, turnips, walnuts
salicylate-free foods	0	bamboo shoots (canned), bananas, beansprouts, beetroot, black eye beans, celery, camomile tea, chickpeas, gin, green cabbage, lima beans, malt vinegar, mung beans, poppy seeds, soy beans, soy sauce, split peas, vodka, whisky

eliminating tartrazine

Some people with asthma are thought to have a hypersensitivity to tartrazine, which can trigger an attack. Those most at risk are people who are also sensitive to aspirin or related salicylates (see pages 48–49). One study found that one in three people (31 percent) with aspirin-sensitive asthma were also sensitive to tartrazine, although in another study the frequency was less at only three percent. If you notice that you develop the classic asthma symptoms of wheezing, chest tightness and shortness of breath when you consume food or drinks containing tartrazine (see the chart below), then eliminating tartrazine from your diet may help to reduce the frequency of your attacks. Tartrazine sensitivity is also suspected of causing other symptoms such as: nausea, nasal congestion, blurred vision, itchy, lumpy skin rash (urticaria), purple skin rash (vasculitis), contact dermatitis, facial swelling (angioedema), migraine, palpitations, behavioural changes (especially anxiety and hyperactivity) and sleep disturbance.

A practitioner will usually diagnose a tartrazine sensitivity when consuming tartrazine-containing products triggers your asthma symptoms. Sometimes a practitioner may give you a test food (such as processed cheese containing artificial food colour), and then monitor your reaction. You should test for a tartrazine sensitivity only under medical supervision.

What is tartrazine?

The colour of food plays an important part in its appeal, which is why both natural colourings and artificial dyes are added to many manufactured and processed

---

Foods containing tartrazine

If you suspect you have a tartrazine sensitivity, it's important to avoid foods that may contain artificial food colours. Some toiletries and cosmetics also contain tartrazine, so use hypo-allergenic products if you are tartrazine sensitive.

check the labels of these foods if you are tartrazine sensitive:

biscuits; breakfast cereals; brown sauce; cakes and cake mixes; cheeses that are processed, such as cheese straws; cream cheese; chewing gum; chocolates; crackers; crisps and savoury snacks; custards and custard powders; ready-made desserts; dips; fizzy drinks and drink mixers; fromage frais; fruit cocktails and cordials; gravy mixes; honey-flavoured products; horseradish; ice creams; jams and marmalades; jellies; ketchups; lemon- and/or lime-flavoured products, for example, cordials; liqueurs; maraschino cherries; margarines; marzipan; milk shakes and flavoured milks; mint sauce/jelly; meal replacement products for slimmers; mustards; pasta meals; pickles; processed meats and fish; salad cream; sauces; smoked cod and haddock; soups; soy sauce; sweets; tinned, processed peas; vegetable juices; vitamin and mineral supplements; yogurts foods. Tartrazine is an artificial, lemon-yellow food dye that is added to many convenience foods. It was originally derived from coal-tar, but is now produced synthetically. On food labels it may appear as FD&C Yellow 5 (in the US) or as additive number E102 (in Europe).

During the 1970s, many cases of tartrazine sensitivity were reported, which led to regulations that required the listing of tartrazine and related dyes on labels. Tartrazine is banned in some countries, such as Norway, and was at one time banned in Austria and Germany too, before EC regulations lifted the ban.

Checking food labels

It's estimated that we each consume around 15mg of artificial dyes every day, of which 85 percent are tartrazine. As well as its use as a yellow colouring agent, tartrazine is mixed with other food dyes to make different colours, such as oranges, browns, blues and a variety of greens. If you're sensitive to tartrazine, it's not enough to avoid yellow-coloured foods. You need to check labels on foods and medicines for FD&C Yellow 5 or E102. Labelling regulations in different countries vary. Tartrazine may appear on labels as "colour" or "artificial colour" if it doesn't have to be specifically indicated by law. Similarly, if tartrazine occurs as a secondary ingredient, such as in the jam within a cake, tartrazine may not have to appear on the label unless the jam contributes more than two percent of the product's weight. In the EU, new laws mean that all major allergens, at any level, must be indicated on the label, but the list of major allergens may vary from country to country. If you're in any doubt, prepare food from raw ingredients.

How does tartrazine cause symptoms?

Consuming too much tartrazine (more than 885mg), triggers the release of histamine from mast cells in the respiratory tract, even in people who don't have a sensitivity. This is a pharmacological, drug-like reaction. However, if you *are* sensitive to tartrazine, you react to much lower amounts – 1mg or less. Although tartrazine triggers histamine release, the mechanism by which it does so doesn't seem to involve the immune system. For this reason, tartrazine sensitivity is not considered to be a true allergic response.

Some people who are sensitive to aspirin and other salicylates (see pages 48–49) are also sensitive to tartrazine, and it's thought that both substances may provoke symptoms in the same way – by blocking the action of COX-1. This enzyme is involved in the breakdown of arachidonic acid, present in all cell membranes. When COX-1 is inhibited, arachidonic acid is broken down to produce increased quantities of inflammatory leukotrienes. These worsen asthma symptoms. Research in this area remains inconclusive.

Turmeric – a natural alternative

Natural yellow food colourings that are used instead of tartrazine include annatto, carotenoids, saffron and turmeric (shown below). These are safe for you to eat.

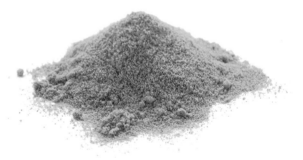

eliminating benzoates

Some people with asthma are hypersensitive to benzoates – when they eat foods containing them, they get an attack. In one study involving 36 people with asthma, significant wheeziness occurred in seven people, five of whom were also sensitive to aspirin. Other studies back up the finding that those who are likely to have a benzoate sensitivity also have an aspirin or salicylate sensitivity. The number of people affected is likely to be small, but if you are among those who are susceptible to benzoates, eliminating them from your diet may help to reduce the frequency of your asthma attacks.

Unbleached flour

Make sure you use unbleached flour (as shown here) if you are sensitive to benzoates; benzoyl peroxide is commonly used as a bleaching agent.

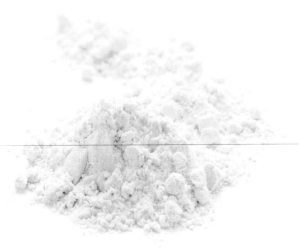

People with a benzoate sensitivity may develop the classic asthma symptoms of wheezing, chest tightness and shortness of breath when they consume food or drinks containing one of this class of preservatives. Benzoate sensitivity can also cause other symptoms such as: itchy, lumpy rash (urticaria), purple skin rash (vasculitis), swelling of the mouth and face (angioedema), nasal inflammation (rhinitis) and headache. Interestingly, a recent study found that eliminating artificial colourings and benzoate preservatives from children's diets produced significant improvements in behaviour, with less hyperactivity. These improvements occurred whether or not the children had asthma.

Sensitivity to benzoates is usually diagnosed by linking asthma symptoms to the consumption of benzoate-containing products. Cinnamon, which has a high natural benzoate content, is sometimes used as a test food to check for benzoate sensitivity. First, however, you have to rule out a salicylate sensitivity as cinnamon also contains a high salicylate content. Using a test food in this way should be carried out only under medical supervision.

If you suspect you have a benzoate sensitivity, it's important to avoid or reduce your intake of foods that may contain these preservatives. You should also avoid over-the-counter acne treatments containing benzoyl peroxide, and anti-dust-mite products that contain benzoate insecticides, such as benzyl benzoate or denatonium benzoate. Some mouthwashes also contain benzoates.

What are benzoates?

Among the most commonly used food additives in the world, benzoates are preservatives that prevent the growth of bacteria, yeasts and fungi in many foods and drinks, especially in those that are acidic. Benzoyl peroxide is also used as a bleaching agent in flours, breads, lecithin and some cheeses, such as soft Italian cheeses, blue cheeses (especially Gorgonzola) and feta cheese. Processed convenience foods such as pies, jams, frozen desserts, sauces, chocolate and confectionery frequently have added benzoates. Around 75 percent of people can detect the taste of sodium benzoate in foods – it's variably perceived as sweet, salty or sometimes bitter. On food labels, benzoates may appear as:

- Benzoic acid
- Sodium benzoate
- Potassium benzoate
- Calcium benzoate
- Ethyl paraben (ethyl para-hydroxybenzoate)
- Sodium ethyl para-hydroxybenzoate
- Propylparaben (propyl para-hydroxybenzoate)
- Sodium propyl para-hydroxybenzoate
- Methyl paraben (methyl para-hydroxybenzoate)
- Sodium methyl para-hydroxybenzoate

When benzoates are used as a food additive, the amount present is usually less than a tenth of a percent by weight. Benzoates also occur naturally in some foods, especially organically grown ones (natural benzoates may occur in greater concentrations than artificially added ones). In particular, berries such as cranberries may have a high benzoic acid content.

How do benzoates cause symptoms?

The way in which benzoates can trigger asthma is unknown, but may involve the production of inflammatory chemicals in a similar way to aspirin and other salicylates (see pages 48–49).

Foods containing benzoates

foods naturally containing benzoates:

anise, apples, avocadoes, black tea, blackberries, blackcurrants, blueberries, cassia bark, cinnamon, cloves, cranberries, greengages, kidney beans, nectarines, nutmeg, peaches, papayas, plums, prunes, pumpkins, raspberries, red beans (such as adzuki beans), redcurrants, soy beans, spinach, strawberries

foods to which benzoates are added as a preservative:

beer; beetroot; bleached flours; caviar; cheeses, especially blue cheeses, Italian soft cheeses and feta cheese; chewing gum; chocolate and confectionery; cider; essences (such as vanilla essence); fish products (such as marinated herrings and soused mackerel); fizzy drinks; flavourings; fruit juices; pulps; purées; pie fillings; ice used to cool fish products; ice creams; jams and marmalades; jellies; ketchups; maraschino cherries; margarine; mincemeats; olives; pickles; prawns; processed meat and fish products; salad dressings; sauces (such as barbecue, chilli, hoisin, oyster and soy); spice mixes; cordials; syrups; vinegars; vinaigrettes; yogurt

eliminating msg

Some people with asthma recognize that consuming monosodium glutamate (MSG) can trigger an asthma attack. In one study involving 32 people with asthma, 14 reacted to MSG, while in another only two out of 30 people experienced respiratory symptoms. Several other studies have found no reactions to MSG even in people with a history of asthma attacks in Chinese restaurants, where high amounts of MSG are typically used during cooking. Some researchers believe these discrepancies are because symptoms may come on only after consuming MSG on an empty stomach, or only with alcohol – these hasten MSG absorption and therefore increase the severity and rate of onset of symptoms. It's also thought that the people who are most sensitive are those with a vitamin-B6 deficiency. There is some evidence that people with an MSG sensitivity stop reacting to it when they take daily vitamin-B6 supplements for at least 12 weeks.

People who have an MSG sensitivity may respond to MSG by getting classic asthma symptoms such as wheezing, chest tightness, shortness of breath and difficulty breathing. MSG sensitivity can also cause non-respiratory symptoms such as: flushing or facial tingling, burning or numbness in the back of the neck and upper body, headache, nausea, shaking, sweating, diarrhea, abdominal pain, palpitations and weakness. If you suspect you have an MSG sensitivity, it's important to avoid all foods that may contain it – see the chart below for a list of foods in which MSG is naturally present or added as a flavour enhancer.

There is no specific test for MSG sensitivity – it is usually diagnosed by the recognition that your asthma symptoms are triggered by consuming MSG-containing products. In people whose asthma is sensitive to MSG, symptoms typically start one to two hours after eating the trigger food. But bear in mind that symptoms may also appear up to 12 hours later.

Foods containing MSG

foods naturally containing MSG:	commonly added as a flavour enhancer to:
kombu seaweed (this has an exceptionally high content of glutamate), tomatoes, mushrooms and cheese	beef stock, biscuits, cereals, chicken stock, Chinese dishes, crackers, crisps, croutons, cured and processed meats, flavouring mixes, freeze-dried foods, frozen foods, gravy and gravy powders, herbal seasoning mixes, instant noodles, Japanese dishes, microwave dinners, pickles, ready meals (especially pasta, pizza, rice and noodle dishes), restaurant meals, salads, dressings and mayonnaises, sauces, smoked meats, snacks, soups and soup mixes, spice mixes, stock cubes and powders, take-aways, vegetables (canned), yeast extract

In people whose asthma is sensitive to MSG, symptoms typically start one to two hours after eating the trigger food. But bear in mind that symptoms may also appear up to 12 hours later.

What is MSG?

MSG is an amino-acid flavour enhancer used especially in Asian cuisine. Sensitivity to MSG is sometimes described as "Chinese restaurant syndrome" although MSG is by no means unique to Chinese food (see the box on the opposite page). MSG stimulates specific taste bud receptors to induce a savoury or meaty taste known in Japan as *umami*. This taste is now accepted as one of the five basic tastes along with saltiness, sweetness, sourness and bitterness. This flavour enhancer was first discovered by extracting crystals of glutamic acid (glutamate) from a broth made from kombu seaweed.

MSG may be listed on food labels by its full name monosodium glutamate, but it also sometimes appears as the following:

- Sodium glutamate
- 2-aminoglutaric acid
- E621 (in the European Union)
- Hydrolyzed vegetable protein (HVP)
- Hydrolyzed plant protein (HPP)
- "Natural flavour"

People who are highly sensitive to MSG may also react to other glutamic acid salts. The names to check for and avoid are:

- Glutamic acid
- Monopotassium glutamate
- Monoammonium glutamate
- Magnesium diglutamate

How does MSG cause symptoms?

Consuming MSG increases blood levels of the amino acid glutamate. This acts as a building block for making the neurotransmitter acetylcholine, which is believed to trigger asthma symptoms.

superfoods for asthma

The following foods are especially helpful for people with asthma. Some contain omega-3 fatty acids that reduce the production of inflammatory substances in the body; some contain antioxidants that reduce inflammatory reactions; while others have a direct effect on your airways to reduce constriction and promote dilation so you can breathe more easily. Although these foods have been identified as general superfoods for asthma, some people have idiosyncratic reactions that mean these foods actually *trigger* asthma. Also, workers in some industries may develop occupational asthma (see page 14) as a result of inhaling allergens found in shellfish, green coffee beans and cocoa beans. Always avoid foods that you think – or have been told – worsen your asthma, especially if you are sensitive to salicylates (see pages 48–49).

superfood	respiratory benefits	how to use it
apples A rich source of powerful antioxidants, such as quercetin, which reduces histamine release and promotes bronchial relaxation.	People who eat five or more apples per week have significantly better lung function than non-apple eaters. Eating apples during pregnancy may protect offspring from asthma.	Eat an apple a day. Grate and add to salads, coleslaw or breakfast cereals (mix with lemon juice to prevent browning). Also snack on dried apple rings or apple crisps.
bananas These are rich in vitamin B6 and a good source of vitamin C, potassium and magnesium.	Children who eat bananas at least once a day are a third less likely to have asthma than those eating bananas less than once a month.	Eat as a snack; slice them onto cereal, into yogurt, or add to low-fat custard. They are delicious added to curries, or barbecued in their skins.
blackcurrants One of the richest fruit sources of antioxidant anthocyanins. They have a strong anti-inflammatory action and also inhibit viral and bacterial growth.	The high ORAC (oxygen radical absorbance capacity) of blackcurrants suggests they can damp down airway inflammation.	Purée to make a coulis; add to smoothies; mix with other berries and serve with low-fat yogurt or fromage frais.
blueberries These berries have one of the highest antioxidant scores of all fruits.	May protect against oxidation in the lungs and circulation.	Eat them fresh, dried, frozen or cooked. Use in smoothies or serve as a coulis with low-fat frozen yogurt.
brazil nuts The richest dietary source of antioxidant selenium – a single brazil nut contains around 50mcg. Also a good source of magnesium.	Those with the highest dietary intake of selenium are more than 40 percent less likely to have asthma than those with the lowest intake.	Eat as a snack, or chop and scatter over cereal, yogurts or salad. Brazil nut butter is a delicious spread.
camomile tea This contains anti-allergenic and anti-inflammatory substances.	Reduces histamine release and nocturnal cough. May also protect against colds.	Have a cup of camomile tea at night before retiring – camomile also promotes calm and sleep.

superfood	respiratory benefits	how to use it
carrots A rich source of antioxidant carotenoids, such as betacarotene, and a good source of vitamin C.	Children with the highest intakes of betacarotene are up to 20 percent less likely to develop asthma than those with low intakes.	Eat raw with dips; grate in salads or in sandwiches. Steam to accompany meat and fish dinners. Purple carrots may offer even more protection.
cherries Provide antioxidant quercetin and anthocyanidins, with the highest quantities found in black cherries. A good source of vitamin C.	People with high intakes of quercetin-rich foods, including fresh cherries, have a lower risk of asthma.	Purée and pour over frozen yogurt or other desserts. Juice cherries and dilute with apple juice. Stone and dip into melted dark chocolate.
chocolate A rich source of flavonoids – gram for gram, dark chocolate has five times more antioxidant activity than blueberries. Also contains theobromine, a bronchodilator.	Dark chocolate is a powerful cough-suppressant, even more effective than codeine, which is a component of over-the-counter cough medicines. An edible spacer device, made from chocolate, was found to improve the bronchodilator effect of reliever inhalers in children!	Eat 50–100g of dark (at least 70 percent cocoa solids) chocolate daily, unless you are watching your weight. Or grate chocolate into hot milk. Unsweetened cocoa is beneficial, too.
coffee A source of methylxanthines, such as caffeine, which act as bronchodilators.	Regular coffee intake reduces the chance of asthma symptoms by 30 percent compared with not drinking coffee. Three to six cups a day can reduce the number of asthma attacks and improve exercise-induced asthma.	Drink three to four cups of coffee per day (more than this may cause tremors, sleep problems and withdrawal symptoms). Ground coffee provides more benefit than instant coffee.
dark green leafy vegetables A good source of antioxidant carotenoids, vitamin C and the anti-spasmodic mineral magnesium – especially broccoli, spring greens, dark green cabbage and parsley.	Women with the highest intake of dark green leafy vegetables are 18 percent less likely to have asthma than those with the lowest intakes.	Steam lightly to accompany meals. Use raw baby spinach leaves in salads. Add green leaves to the mix when juicing fruit and vegetables.
elderberries A rich source of antioxidant anthocyanins. Also contain powerful antiviral agents that protect against coughs, colds and influenza.	Elderberry juice can shorten the duration of a cold or influenza by up to four days. Its antioxidants reduce inflammation and may reduce wheeze.	Make home-made elderberry jam or wine. Add berries to summer puddings, cereals and yogurts. You can also take an elderberry supplement.
garlic A source of allicin – a powerful antioxidant.	Garlic has antibacterial and antiviral properties, and stimulates the immune system. Garlic reduces susceptibility to colds and also shortens their severity and duration.	Use in all savoury dishes. Add toward the end of cooking for maximum benefits.

superfood	respiratory benefits	how to use it
guava Contains four to 10 times as much vitamin C as oranges (the peel is a very good source). Pink guava has a high lycopene content.	Lycopene can protect against exercise-induced asthma. (People with asthma tend to have low intakes of lycopene.)	Eat pink guava for breakfast or as a dessert. Use guava peel as well as the flesh for maximum vitamin C when making purées or juices.
ginger Contains volatile oils such as gingerols, shogaols and gingerdiols.	Ginger reduces inflammation, has an antiviral action, loosens phlegm and acts as an expectorant.	Drink ginger tea and dry ginger ale. Add ginger to desserts, curries, soups and stews.
grape juice Black/purple grapes have a high antioxidant score. Red grape juice provides similar benefits to red wine.	Children eating the most grapes are least likely to develop wheezing or rhinitis.	Drink grape juice on its own or mixed with other juices. Use as the liquid in fresh fruit salad and jellies. Avoid grape juice with added sulfites.
mango A rich source of antioxidant carotenoids, and vitamins C and E.	Increasing carotenoid intake can relieve asthma symptoms. May reduce bronchospasm.	Eat fresh in fruit salads or on its own. Use in fruit coulis, shakes and smoothies.
milk A good source of protein, calcium and B vitamins.	A study of 1,600 adults found those drinking milk had a 34 percent lower risk of asthma symptoms than those not drinking milk.	Use it on cereals, and in drinks, smoothies, shakes and milk puddings.
mustard Mustard seeds are an Ayurvedic treatment for asthma. Those who are sensitive to salicylates should avoid mustard.	Contains substances that help to dampen inflammation.	Add mustard seeds to curries, stews and soups. Use sprouted mustard seeds in salads. Steam mustard greens lightly.
oily fish A rich source of anti-inflammatory omega-3 fatty acids (EPA and DHA), which limit leukotriene synthesis. Also contain antioxidant vitamins A and E.	People who eat oily fish at least twice a week are half as likely to experience asthma, wheezing or chest tightness on waking compared to those who eat little oily fish. Fish oils reduce the severity of exercise-induced asthma.	Eat two to four portions of oily fish a week. Steam, grill or bake fresh fish, or eat sushi and sashimi. Girls and women should limit their intake to two portions a week (as sea pollutants, such as mercury, may affect the health of future offspring).
olive oil A rich source of monounsaturated fats, and antioxidant, anti-inflammatory substances.	Children following a Mediterranean-style diet that includes olive oil are less likely to develop wheezing, rhinitis and other allergic symptoms.	Use olive oil as your standard cooking oil. Use extra virgin olive oil in salad dressings and for drizzling on food, and with bread.
onions A rich source of flavonoid antioxidants. Thiosulfinates isolated from onions have a powerful anti-inflammatory action.	Eating onions five or more times a week reduces the risk of asthma symptoms by 25 percent.	Make French onion soup. Serve onion sauces and onion marmalade with meat. Slice raw red onions into salads (they are high in antioxidants).

superfood	respiratory benefits	how to use it
pears Contain pectins and bioflavonoids that suppress allergic responses (especially Asian pears). Pears rarely trigger allergies and are important in elimination diets.	Adolescents with the highest intake of pears are 17 percent less likely to have asthma than those with the lowest intake.	Eat raw pears as a snack. Poach pears in red wine. Add to fruit salads. Juice pears and combine with apple or grape juice.
pomegranate A rich source of antioxidant polyphenols, anthocyanins, vitamins C and E and carotenoids. Its antioxidant potential is two or three times higher than that of red wine and green tea.	Pomegranate juice has an anti-inflammatory action that can reduce asthma symptoms such as wheezing. It also has a powerful antiviral and antibacterial action against infections.	Look for fresh pomegranate juice drinks, or juice your own. Add pomegranate seeds to salads and desserts.
red wine A rich source of antioxidant polyphenols.	People drinking three to five glasses of red wine per week have a 30 percent lower risk of asthma than non-drinkers.	Have one to two glasses, once or twice a week if wine does not worsen your asthma. Select wines with no added sulfites (some natural sulfites will remain).
teas White, green, oolong and black teas contain high levels of flavonoid catechins, such as epigallocatechin-3-gallate (EGCG) and gallic acid, plus methylxanthines, such as caffeine and theobromine, and small amounts of theophylline (an anti-asthma drug first extracted from tea leaves).	EGCG has anti-allergy properties. Gallic acid has antioxidant, anti-inflammatory and antimicrobial actions. Theophylline is a powerful bronchodilator. Theanine, an amino acid in tea, promotes relaxation. Two to three cups a day can reduce the risk of asthma by 28 percent.	Drink green, black or white tea regularly, three to five times a day. Use left-over cold tea to soak dried fruit, as a basis for sauces, soups or stews, or to make ice cream.
tomatoes A rich source of the red carotenoid lycopene. Cooking releases more lycopene for absorption.	The benefits are the same as eating guava, which is also rich in lycopene.	Make tomato-based sauces, stews and soups. Serve roast tomatoes with fish and meats. Drink tomato juice.
turmeric Has a powerful anti-inflammatory action equivalent to that of some corticosteroids.	Dilates the airways (the more you eat, the better). Relieves cough. Reduces mucus production.	Add to curries, soups and stews. Use to colour rice dishes and desserts. Drink tea made from turmeric root.
walnuts A rich source of omega-3 fatty acids.	Children who eat nuts at least three times a week are half as likely to wheeze than those with a low intake.	Add chopped walnuts to cereals, salads, vegetarian dishes and desserts. Use walnut butter as a spread.
yogurt Live bio-yogurts contain probiotic bacteria, which prime the immune system against allergic responses.	When taken during pregnancy, and/or given to infants, probiotics can reduce the incidence of allergic conditions such as asthma.	Eat live bio-yogurt with breakfast cereals, and with chopped fruit as a dessert. Drink probiotic drinks.

supplements for asthma

These are the supplements that I recommend for people with asthma. Although diet should always come first, many people don't get all the vitamins and minerals they need from food. When you have an inflammatory condition such as asthma, your need for antioxidants is increased, and I believe it's impossible to consistently achieve the high level of antioxidant protection you need from diet alone. There are no miracle cures, but many supplements can reduce inflammation, promote airway relaxation and improve symptoms. Supplements are widely available in pharmacies and healthfood stores. Unless I mention otherwise, they are best taken after food for maximum absorption and to reduce possible side effects such as indigestion – just four bites of food will do. Don't take supplements during pregnancy or breastfeeding except under the advice of a medical herbalist or experienced nutritional therapist. If taking prescribed medications, check with a pharmacist for any potential interactions. Always keep supplements out of the reach of children.

supplement	research findings	dose and comment
vitamin C A powerful antioxidant that protects the airways and reduces inflammation triggered by inhaled antigens. Also reduces the release of histamine and protects against colds.	Can reduce asthma attacks; reduce the dose of corticosteroids needed to control asthma; and protect against exercise-induced asthma when taken 30 minutes before exertion.	500–2,000mg a day, preferably in two divided doses. Avoid indigestion with high doses by taking non-acidic ester-C.
vitamin E A powerful antioxidant that improves immune function.	Increased intake is associated with a reduced incidence of asthma.	200–800mg a day. Select natural source tocopherols.
vitamin B6 Blood levels of this vitamin are lower in people with asthma.	Reduces the frequency and severity of wheezing in some. Important for those taking theophylline, which depletes B6 levels further.	50mg, twice a day.
vitamin B12 Essential for blood cell production and DNA synthesis.	Binds with sulfites and can protect against sulfite-induced asthma.	1–1.5mg per week as a sublingual tablet.
lycopene An antioxidant carotenoid found in tomatoes.	Protects against exercise-related asthma in some people.	10–30mg a day.
magnesium Blood levels are lower in people with asthma.	Inhibits airway constriction. Relieves asthma symptoms.	300–750mg a day.
selenium Needed for the formation of powerful antioxidant enzymes (glutathione peroxidases).	Lowered activity of glutathione peroxidase enzymes is linked with aspirin-induced asthma.	50–200mcg selenium a day.

the natural health approach

supplement	research findings	dose and comment
omega-3 fish oils Eicosapentaenoic acid (EPA) and docosahexaenoic acid (DHA) reduce production of inflammatory chemicals.	Reduce the severity of asthma symptoms and reduce bronchial reactivity. Protect against exercise-induced asthma.	500mg–5g a day.
green-lipped mussel Raw extracts have an anti-inflammatory action to reduce production of leukotrienes.	Significantly reduces daytime wheeze.	350–500mg, three times a day.
quercetin A flavonoid antioxidant that can inhibit the release of histamine. Has a relaxant effect on smooth muscle cells in the airways.	Laboratory research shows it stabilizes airway cells and promotes bronchial relaxation.	500mg, three times a day. Best taken half an hour before food.
n-acetyl-l-cysteine (NAC) An antioxidant amino acid that thins excess mucus and inhibits activity of the white blood cells involved in allergic inflammatory responses.	Reduces the release of inflammatory chemicals and acts as an expectorant by stimulating mechanisms designed to clear mucus from the airways.	100–500mg, three times a day.
co-enzyme Q10 (CoQ10) Needed for oxygen utilization.	When combined with vitamins C and E, can reduce dose of corticosteroids needed to control asthma symptoms.	100–500mg, three times a day.
probiotics Prime the immune system with "friendly" bacteria to reduce the development of allergic diseases.	Inhibit airway hypersensitivity and allergic airway response. Taking during pregnancy and in infancy may protect against childhood asthma.	1–5 billion live bacteria (colony forming units or CFU) per dose.
pycnogenol Extracts from the bark of the French maritime pine contain a powerful array of antioxidants. As effective in preventing release of histamine as sodium cromoglicate (see page 19).	Reduces frequency and severity of asthma symptoms. Reduces the need for inhalers. Can block 70 percent of histamine release from mast cells when they are exposed to airborne allergens such as pollen.	50mg–200mg a day.
reishi A Chinese mushroom with antioxidant, anti-inflammatory, antiviral and antibacterial properties.	Reduces production of inflammatory chemicals in the airways. Reduces bronchial hypersensitivity.	500mg, once, twice or three times a day.
digestive enzymes Increases stomach-acid production.	Boosts breakdown of high protein foods to reduce intolerances that make asthma worse. Pepsin, betaine and glutamic acid increase stomach acid production, which may reduce asthma symptoms (see pages 14–15).	1 to 4 capsules a day. Take at the start of a meal. Select a broad spectrum complex that contains a mixture of plant-derived proteases, such as bromelain and papain.

lifestyle approaches to treatment

Lifestyle changes that minimize your exposure to trigger factors, such as house dust mites and pollen, are just as important in your asthma management as medication – prevention really is better than cure. Try to work out what triggers your attacks so you can avoid these factors (see pages 63–65 for detailed advice).

If you are overweight, I strongly recommend that you try to lose weight. A recent study involving more than 3,000 adults suggests that those who were overweight or obese were more likely to have persistent and severe asthma, and less likely to enjoy regular periods of remission. Overall, those who were obese were 66 percent more likely to report continuous symptoms and 36 percent more likely to miss more than two days off work per year owing to asthma than normal-weight adults with asthma. See pages 66–67 to find out if you are overweight and to discover sustainable ways to lose weight if you are.

Taking up regular exercise and quitting smoking can also have remarkably beneficial effects on your respiratory health – as both of these can pose a considerable challenge, I explain how to make these lifestyle changes in manageable ways on pages 68–71.

Managing stress

Anger, stress or joy can all trigger asthma. Children often cough when they're excited, while adults may find their asthma flares up before a job interview or after a row. Stress doesn't cause asthma, but it may make the underlying condition worse.

If you know that stress exacerbates your asthma, find stress-relief techniques that work for you. Try therapies such as yoga, aromatherapy, meditation, visualization and self-massage. During moments of stress, concentrate on breathing slowly (see pages 38–39) so that you don't get into a cycle of overbreathing, which can trigger a panic attack.

During periods of stress at work, look after your general health – don't rely on multiple cups of coffee or cigarettes to get you through the day. Too much coffee mimics the body's stress response and can make you feel panicky, and smoking will make your asthma worse. Learn to be assertive and to say no to extra work. If the pressure is building, remove yourself from a situation and go for a brisk walk – exercise is a great stress-reliever. Or, if you can, go somewhere private and shout as loudly as you can, or punch a soft cushion as hard as possible.

Speleotherapy

Spending time in subterranean caves or salt mines is an accepted therapeutic measure for asthma in some central and Eastern European countries. Called speleotherapy, and sometimes halotherapy or Radon therapy, the technique relies upon a natural environment that's free from common dusts and pollen. Increased levels of carbon dioxide may also play a role in the apparent effectiveness of this strategy (see the Buteyko method, pages 38–39). Using a crystalline rock salt lamp may provide some of the beneficial effects of speleotherapy.

avoiding triggers

Below are many of the culprits responsible for triggering asthma attacks. For each one I describe how best you can avoid it or – where avoidance is impossible – how to minimize your exposure to it or lessen its impact on your lungs.

Avoid pollen

If pollen triggers your asthma, take the simple measure of staying indoors with the windows closed when pollen forecasts are high, especially during thundery weather. If it's essential to go out, apply petroleum jelly (Vaseline) or cellulose powder (Nasaleze) inside your nose to reduce the impact of pollen. Wear sunglasses to minimize eye symptoms. The best times to go out are late morning or early afternoon – pollen counts peak between seven and nine in the morning and again between three and seven in the afternoon and evening. If possible, stay at ground level – pollen rises into the atmosphere, so your symptoms may be worse if you work at the top of a skyscraper, for example.

Keep windows closed when travelling by car, and consider buying a car with an integral pollen filter. If possible, change your clothes and shower after going outside, and wash your hands before touching your eyes. Similarly, avoid pets that have been outdoors and carry pollen on their fur, and don't hang clothes outdoors to dry as pollen will cling to them. Make sure your bedroom windows are closed in the early evening so you don't sleep in a pollen trap at night.

Get rid of house dust mites

Depending on how severe your allergy is, consider replacing wall-to-wall carpets with vinyl floor coverings and washable rugs, and install vertical blinds instead of curtains. Remove books and ornaments that are likely to attract dust, and when you dust, use a damp cloth that collects rather than scatters dust particles. Using a vacuum fitted with an anti-allergy HEPA (high efficiency particulate air) filter removes virtually all airborne particles so they are not blown back out in the vacuum exhaust. Open doors and windows when vacuuming so that dust can escape.

Take special care of bed linen, pillows and mattresses: when changing sheets, avoid shaking them; vacuum mattresses and pillows once a week (or use mattress and pillow anti-allergen barriers designed to seal mites in). Wash all bedding at least once a week at 60°C to kill mites. Avoid drying washing indoors, where possible, as this increases humidity, which needs to be kept below 45 percent to prevent house dust mites flourishing. Use a condenser-style clothes drier, and a room dehumidifier if necessary.

If your child has asthma, don't let him or her sleep on a bottom bunk – they'll be in close proximity to two mattresses. Instead put them on the top bunk, or in a separate bed if you can. Remove allergens from

Invest in an ionizer

An air ionizer is a relatively inexpensive device that can reduce levels of airborne particles such as pollen, dust, smoke, bacteria, viruses, mould spores and animal allergens by releasing negatively charged ions. These collide with suspended particles, which carry a positive electrical charge, causing them to clump together and fall out of the air. Negative ions also seem to neutralize the adverse respiratory effects of dust and pollen. Use a negative ionizer in your bedroom, living room and in your workspace. You can also use some models in cars.

favourite cuddly toys by placing them in the freezer overnight, then washing them at 60°C once a week.

Anti-dust mite sprays are useful, but note that some people may be sensitive to the chemicals in them.

Get rid of fungal spores and moulds

Keeping the humidity level low (below 45 percent) in your home is the most important step toward reducing fungi and moulds, which tend to thrive in warm, humid environments. Use an air conditioner in summer, and a heater in winter. Ventilate the kitchen and bathroom well, and frequently inspect tiles, shower curtains, windows and ceilings for signs of mould growth, and regularly wipe them down with an antifungal solution. Don't leave fruit and bread lying around as these rapidly turn mouldy. Empty and clean bins regularly. House-dust-mite avoidance measures also help (see page 63), as the mould *Aspergillus repens*, is closely associated with dust mites. Don't enter damp basements or rooms that are poorly ventilated, and avoid decomposing leaves, grasses and grains (for example, don't rake garden leaves). Wear an industrial mask if exposure to moulds is an occupational hazard.

Limit your risk of viral infections

Viruses are to blame for 80 percent of episodes of reduced peak flow or wheezing. Unfortunately, the common cold virus is highly infectious and spreads readily through airborne droplets from coughs and sneezes. To limit your risk of infection, eat a healthy diet, avoid excess stress and get plenty of sleep to boost your natural immunity. Avoid smoky atmospheres, which damage airways and make infection more likely. Avoid people with obvious cold symptoms (in particular, don't shake hands with them). Wash your hands regularly, and use antibacterial hand wipes or sprays for extra protection; and use antiviral tissues to kill cold viruses (viruses can survive for at least 24 hours in standard tissues). Consider taking vitamin-C supplements which may reduce the duration and severity of a cold (and help your asthma). Ask your doctor about receiving an annual influenza vaccination.

Avoid animal fur and feathers

If your pets trigger your asthma, make sure someone washes them at least once a week when you're not around, to reduce the amount of allergen they shed. Try to limit the animals to a designated part of the house, and never let them into your bedroom.

Traditionally it was believed that synthetic pillows were better than feather pillows for people with asthma, as they do not contain animal proteins. However, recent research suggests that feather pillows may actually be better for people with asthma than synthetic ones, as they harbor significantly less cat, dog and dust mite allergens. People using non-feather pillows suffer more frequent episodes of wheezing than those using feather pillows. Select a traditional feather pillow covered with a special waterproof, semi-permeable membrane that allows your skin to breathe, while keeping out dust mites and bacteria.

Minimize exposure to cigarette smoke

Second-hand smoking of both sidestream smoke (smoke that wafts from burning tobacco) and mainstream smoke (exhaled by a smoker) exposes you to lung irritants such as:

- Carbon monoxide – a poisonous gas also found in exhaust fumes.
- Tar – used for surfacing roads.
- Nicotine – an effective pesticide.
- Acetone – used as a paint and varnish stripper.
- Ammonia – a scouring cleaning agent.
- Poisons such as arsenic, benzene, cadmium, formaldehyde, hydrogen cyanide and methanol.

Other people's smoke is a common trigger for asthma and damages your airways so that viruses and bacteria can enter more easily. Avoid smoky atmospheres, and don't let anyone smoke in your home or car. Don't rely on air conditioners to eliminate smoke – they don't remove dangerous micro-particles. For advice about quitting smoking, go to pages 70–71.

Protect yourself from chemicals at work

Avoid exposure to dangerous chemicals and chemical sensitizers at work wherever possible. If this isn't feasible, reduce your contact to the lowest possible level. Wear protective clothing, including a face mask, or work in an area fitted with extractor fans. Persuade your workplace to restrict smoking to designated areas or ban it altogether (this is now a legal requirement in many countries). Use your preventer inhaler regularly – ask your doctor or asthma nurse to check that your technique is good, and that you are on the right dose. Discuss asthma symptoms with your occupational nurse or doctor, and be sure to inform your workplace's health-and-safety representative of any problems.

Stay out of cold or damp air

Breathing in cold air triggers asthma in some people, while others experience tightness and wheezing when moving from a cold environment into the warm. Limit outdoor activity when it is very cold and wet – spend more time indoors. If you need to go outside, dress warmly and cover your mouth and nose with a scarf. If you suspect weather conditions are likely to bring on your asthma, use your reliever inhaler five to 10 minutes before going outside.

Protect yourself from air pollution

Traffic fumes – especially from diesel engines, which emit 10 times as many particles as petrol engines – are a powerful asthma trigger. Poor air quality owing to a

Choose low-allergen holidays

If you have pollen-sensitive asthma, take your holiday by the seaside rather than deep in the country – sea breezes help to keep pollen grains inland. Pollen counts are often three times higher in continental Europe than in the UK, but on-shore winds mean the west coast of Europe is relatively clear of pollen, as are the Mediterranean islands. Alpine resorts in Switzerland and Austria are usually suitable for people with asthma, too. If you plan to visit Europe, go during August or September, when the worst pollen season is over. Also avoid hot, humid environments if these bring on symptoms, and consider visiting a low-allergen area such as Arad, in Israel, west of the Dead Sea. Arad is specifically designed to provide an environment free from pollution and allergenic pollens – garden plantings are carefully controlled. When travelling abroad always make sure you take enough anti-asthma medication with you. And carry your inhaler with you on the plane in case you need it.

build up of gases such as nitrogen oxides and low-lying ozone also makes asthma worse. If you go out in poor-quality air, wear a face mask with an integral air filter – cotton or silk versions are available. These are especially useful when cycling or walking near traffic.

Find alternatives to volatile chemicals

Volatile chemicals in solvents, paint, polishes, glues, air fresheners and perfumes can trigger asthma in some people. If this applies to you, look for alternatives. For example, when decorating your home, use water-based paints (emulsions) instead of oil-based paints. And rather than wearing perfume, use an essential-oil blend diluted with carrier oil (see page 25).

maintaining a healthy weight

Obesity and asthma are both conditions that are associated with increased levels of inflammatory chemicals in the body. It's therefore not surprising that being overweight or obese increases the chance of having asthma, and also increases its severity. Being overweight also affects how well your medication can control your asthma. The good news is that people who lose excess weight can significantly reduce the frequency and severity of their asthma symptoms.

What's your ideal weight?

The easiest way to see if you are in the ideal weight range for your height is to use the chart on the opposite page. Look for the point on the lines where your weight and height intersect. If the point falls in the yellow zone, you are in the ideal weight range for your height. If it falls in the orange or red zones, then losing some excess fat could improve your asthma. And if it falls in the white zone, you are underweight and could benefit from putting on weight. Some research shows that, for men in particular, being underweight can make your asthma worse.

How to lose weight

The best way to lose weight is to permanently change your eating habits, so you eat more healthily without feeling you're actually on a diet. As well as eating less, it helps to do more exercise. Small changes in your approach to food can also help; for example, pause during meals so they last longer and your body has time to fill up before you've overeaten. And don't eat everything on your plate out of habit.

Five main types of weight-loss diet exist, each with their proponents and detractors:

- Low-calorie diets, which provide 1,000–1,500 kcals a day, and can help you achieve an average weight loss of 6.5kg (14lb) over six months. However, weight is often regained within one year.
- Low-fat diets, which restrict total fat intake to less than 30 percent of your energy intake. After six months, average weight loss is 5.1kg (11lb), but weight is usually regained within one year.
- Very low-calorie diets, which provide 400–800 kcals a day in the form of fortified, sweet or savoury meal-replacement drinks. These are followed under close professional supervision and can help you lose between 13–23kg (29–51lb) a year.
- Low-carbohydrate diets, which restrict intake of carbohydrate and concentrate on high-protein foods. These curb appetite and reduce insulin production – the body's main fat-storing hormone. You may lose around 6kg (13lb) over six months.
- Low-glycemic-index diets, which also restrict carbohydrate intake, but not so severely.

There is little evidence that either low-calorie or low-fat diets are effective long-term. Using a very low-calorie diet produces quick results, and has been shown to significantly improve lung function and peak flow in people with asthma. However, you should follow this form of diet only under supervision. Those willing to lose weight more steadily will benefit from either a low-carbohydrate diet or a low-glycemic-index diet. The latter is less controversial; in fact, there's a growing consensus that a low-glycemic diet that emphasizes healthy fats, such as olive oil and omega-3 fish oils, is the diet of choice for overweight people with an inflammatory condition such as asthma. A low-glycemic diet also helps to maintain weight loss.

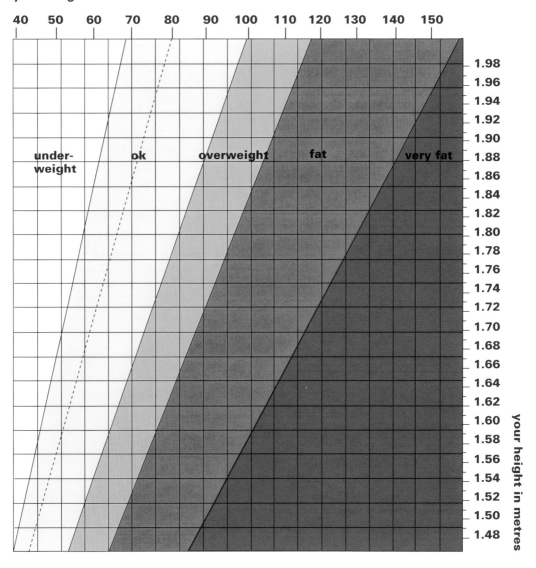

your weight in kilos

| 40 | 50 | 60 | 70 | 80 | 90 | 100 | 110 | 120 | 130 | 140 | 150 |

under-weight   ok   overweight   fat   very fat

your height in metres

1.98
1.96
1.94
1.92
1.90
1.88
1.86
1.84
1.82
1.80
1.78
1.76
1.74
1.72
1.70
1.68
1.66
1.64
1.62
1.60
1.58
1.56
1.54
1.52
1.50
1.48

taking regular exercise

In the long term, regular exercise can relieve asthma by helping you to breathe more efficiently and by strengthening your respiratory muscles. But, in the short term, many people with asthma find that exercise can bring on a fit of coughing, shortness of breath, or wheezing – exercise is the second most common asthma trigger after the common cold. Exactly why exercise induces asthma is not fully understood, but evaporation of water and excessive dryness of the airways is involved. Exercise also increases circulating levels of immune cells, and increases the production of inflammatory chemicals such as leukotrienes and histamine. Long periods of exercise, such as marathon running, are more likely to cause wheezing than short or less vigorous activities, such as a fitness class, swimming or yoga. If you find normal amounts of exercise bring on your symptoms, it suggests your asthma isn't well controlled – seek advice from your doctor or asthma nurse.

What type of exercise?

Physical activity doesn't need to be vigorous and can include activities such as DIY, gardening, dancing and sex, as well as conventional exercise such as walking, swimming or cycling. Prolonged aerobic exercise, such as running or playing football, netball or hockey, is more likely to trigger asthma symptoms than are weightlifting, playing golf or moderate-paced walking. Although swimming is aerobic, the humidity associated with swimming pools means your airways are less likely to react (unless you are sensitive to chlorine). Aim to exercise for at least 30 minutes, five times a week.

How intense?

Exercise doesn't have to be vigorous, but you should pursue less intense forms of exercise for longer to obtain maximum cardiovascular benefits. The chart on the opposite page shows how long you need to exercise at moderate intensity to increase your energy output by 200 kcals per day – enough to slowly lose excess weight and become fit. If you find that exercising for longer than 15 minutes brings on your asthma symptoms, then exercise for two 15-minute sessions or three 10-minute sessions over the course of a day.

Exercise physiologists now realize that interval training, in which you alternate short bursts of high-intensity exercise with gentle recovery during your workout regime can dramatically improve your level of cardiovascular fitness and your body's ability to burn excess fat. For example, sprinting for 30 seconds, and then either stopping or jogging gently for four minutes can double your usual exercise endurance, increase the amount of fat you burn per hour by 36 percent and increase your cardiovascular fitness by 13 percent after only two weeks of changing your usual routine – even in people who are already fairly fit.

Preventing exercise-related asthma

If exercise regularly triggers your asthma, the following tips may help.

- Breathe through your nose as much as you can while exercising to humidify air before it reaches your lungs.

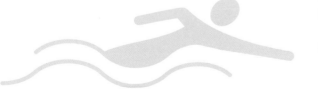

How long it takes to burn 200 kcals

activity	average number of calories burned/hour	time to burn 200 kcals
walking (stroll)	200	1 hour
bowling	250	48 mins
gardening	250	48 mins
gentle love-making	300	40 mins
golf	350	34 mins
swimming	350	34 mins
brisk walking	350	34 mins
dancing	400	30 mins
tennis	500	24 mins
jogging	500	24 mins
vigorous love-making	500	24 mins
cycling	600	20 mins

● Use a reliever inhaler 15 minutes before exercise. This can prevent symptoms for around four hours. It's effective for 80 percent of people with exercise-induced asthma, but if used daily, its effectiveness declines, and if exercise-induced asthma does occur, a second dose is less likely to work.

● If you're doing a longer, more strenuous workout, it's important to warm up properly to prepare your lungs. Doing several 30-second sprints over a five-to-10 minute period seems to condition your lungs and protect against exercise-induced asthma for around 40 minutes. You can also prepare yourself for a long exercise session, such as a tennis game, by cycling briskly for 15 to 30 minutes beforehand.

● Some people find their asthma is exercise-induced only if they're also exposed to another trigger, such as cold air, pollen, mould spores or fumes. If this applies to you, take appropriate action. For example, avoid exercising outside on cold days or when the pollen count is high (especially if it's also thundery). Stay away from areas that are damp and enclosed, such as poorly ventilated basement gyms or dank woodland areas (especially during the peak mushroom season). Avoid exercising near traffic fumes or, if this is impossible, wear a face mask. Exercising in relatively high humidity can help, as long as ventilation is good, such as in a swimming pool, or by a sun-lit lake or stream.

● Don't exercise when you have a respiratory infection – your airways will already be inflamed.

● Take vitamin C and fish oils – research shows that they can protect against exercise-induced asthma (see pages 60–61).

● Cut back on your salt intake – excessive consumption of sodium chloride promotes water retention, which worsens lung congestion.

● If you keep experiencing problems, another treatment option is a mast cell stabilizer, such as cromoglycate or nedocromil. This can prevent symptoms for four hours when used 15 to 60 minutes before exercise – ask your doctor. He or she may also suggest a long-acting bronchodilator, such as salmeterol or formoterol, which can relieve symptoms for up to 12 hours when taken 30 minutes before exercise. Another option is a leukotriene modifier, such as montelukast or zafirlukast, whose actions last for up to 24 hours.

quitting smoking

Smoking is a powerful trigger for asthma. For example, adolescents who regularly smoke at least seven cigarettes per day are four times more likely to develop asthma than non-smokers. Inhaling second-hand smoke can also trigger asthma – people exposed to involuntary passive smoking for more than eight hours a day in the workplace are twice as likely to experience wheezing than those in a smoke-free environment. Only a small amount of smoke is needed to trigger bronchospasm; research carried out by Asthma UK shows that tobacco smoke can trigger symptoms in almost 80 percent of people with asthma.

If you have asthma and smoke cigarettes, it's important that you do your utmost to quit. Apart from bringing on asthma symptoms, smoking is now known to make your preventer inhalers less effective at damping down symptoms. But, if you can stop smoking, the good news is that your response to your asthma treatment will improve.

Quitting techniques

Most people who rely on willpower alone find it "fairly or extremely difficult" to quit. Stopping smoking means having to beat a physical addiction to nicotine, as well as the habit of lighting up. Research suggests that you are physically addicted to nicotine if you smoke more than 20 cigarettes per day, inhale the smoke and need to light up first thing in the morning. If you smoke fewer than 20 cigarettes a day, and never usually light up before breakfast, you are more likely to have a psychological dependency. The following methods can help you to break both physical and psychological dependencies.

Nicotine replacement therapy (NRT) This can double your chance of quitting as it gives you a regular nicotine boost to ease the symptoms of withdrawal. And, if you receive behavioural support or counselling from your doctor, a nurse or pharmacist as well as using NRT, you are at least 26 percent more likely to quit than those using NRT alone. NRT is available in a number of formulations including skin patches, chewing gum, inhalers, sprays, and microtabs that dissolve in the mouth.

Gradual reduction method Research has shown that moderate-to-heavy smokers who reduce their consumption before their eventual quit date are more likely to stop smoking successfully. A technique known as the gradual reduction method helps you cut back on your nicotine intake by trapping the nicotine and tar you would otherwise have inhaled. It involves applying drops of a natural food-grade substance (corn syrup) called NicoBloc (www.nicobloc.com) to the filter of your cigarette immediately before smoking. It is typically used over a six-week period to gently wean you off nicotine. In the first week you apply one drop of NicoBloc to each cigarette filter before smoking to trap 33 percent of tar and nicotine; in the second week you apply two drops to each cigarette filter to block up to two thirds of tar and nicotine; from week

Inhale fragrant oils
Inhaling a combination of the following essential oils can help overcome addictions: basil, benzoin, bergamot, clary sage, frankincense, helichrysum, lavender, narcissus, rose otto, spikenard, vetiver and ylang-ylang. See page 25 for information on how to use essential oils.

three onward you use three drops per cigarette to block up to 99 percent of tar and nicotine. People using this method don't seem to compensate by smoking more cigarettes, and the method isn't associated with increased cravings. A trial involving 800 smokers found that after a six-week gradual reduction program, 60 percent successfully stopped smoking without significant withdrawal symptoms. Even those who continued to smoke consumed an average of 11 fewer cigarettes per day after using the gradual reduction method. Relapsers relapsed to significantly fewer cigarettes per day after using the gradual reduction method compared with those who relapsed after stopping abruptly.

Complementary approaches Hypnosis can help one in three smokers quit and is more effective than using willpower alone. Some practitioners use a combination of hypnotherapy and Neuro Linguistic Programming (NLP) for an even greater success rate. Acupuncture helps one in four smokers quit.

Quit plan

If you plan to quit rather than stopping abruptly, you'll have more chance of success. Choose in advance the date you are going to stop smoking – this will allow you time to get into the right frame of mind. The following tips will also help you avoid pitfalls and enhance your chance of quitting successfully.

- Find support – stopping smoking is easier if you do it with a friend or relative who also wants to quit.
- Throw away all your cigarettes, matches, lighters and ashtrays on your quit date.
- Take it one day at a time – keep a chart and tick off each cigarette-free day.
- Find something to occupy your hands such as drawing, painting, knitting, DIY or origami.

Breathe away cravings
Try the following relaxation exercise to overcome nicotine cravings:

- Breathe in deeply through your mouth so your lungs expand as much as possible.
- Hold your breath for three seconds.
- Let all the air out slowly, until your lungs feel completely empty.
- Don't breathe in for a further three seconds.
- Repeat this cycle twice more, so you have breathed in and out slowly three times.
- Return to breathing normally.

- Increase the amount of exercise you take to help curb withdrawal symptoms. Exercise increases the secretion of opium-like endorphins in the brain – these bring feelings of calm and well-being.
- Avoid situations where you used to smoke.
- Learn to say "No thanks, I've quit" or "No thanks, I'm cutting down" … and mean it.

When you have a strong urge to smoke try the following measures:

- Suck on an artificial cigarette or herbal stick (available in pharmacies).
- Chew celery or carrot sticks.
- Eat an apple.
- Clean your teeth with strongly-flavoured toothpaste.
- Go out for a brisk walk, swim, cycle-ride or jog.
- Take a supplement, such as Nicobrevin, designed to reduce nicotine cravings. Supplements containing oat straw (*Avena sativa*) and flower remedies can also help. Ask your pharmacist for advice about available products.

The natural health guru programs

Having explained the medical aspects of asthma in Part One and the natural approaches to treating it in Part Two, this section shows you how to **put all the information into practice in your day-to-day life.** First, I ask you to complete a questionnaire to help pinpoint which program is right for you: the gentle, moderate or full-strength program. Each program lasts for two weeks to a month. **The gentle program** is aimed at people who will benefit from eating **an anti-inflammatory diet** that supplies more of the key nutrients that can damp down lung inflammation; **the moderate program** is designed to exclude dietary sulfites – a common but under-recognized asthma trigger; and **the full-strength program** excludes dietary salicylates. As well as suggesting what to eat over a 14-day period, each program supplies **healthy asthma-friendly recipes,** a breath control routine, and a series of **complementary therapies to try.** I also suggest which vitamin, mineral and herbal supplements to take depending on the program you are following. After completing these programs, you should notice a **significant improvement in your asthma symptoms** and overall well-being.

the natural health guru starting the programs

Most people with asthma are uncertain whether or not their symptoms are linked to eating particular foods. If this is the case for you, then start with the gentle program to see how you respond. It's likely that your asthma will improve simply because you are increasing your intake of antioxidant-rich fruit and vegetables, omega-3 fish oils and other anti-asthma superfoods, while at the same time cutting back on your intake of pro-inflammatory omega-6 vegetable oils such as sunflower and safflower oil, which are widely present in processed foods. These changes are designed to reduce the amount of inflammation in your body, including your lungs.

After repeating the gentle program so that you follow it for one month in total, your symptoms should have significantly improved. If not, then I'd like you to move on to the moderate program. This is designed to reduce your exposure to dietary sulfites and will reveal whether or not your asthma is linked to a sulfite sensitivity (see pages 46–47). If it is, following the moderate program for two weeks should produce a marked improvement in your symptoms. However, if you don't notice an improvement, please move on to the full-strength program. I have designed this to reduce your exposure to dietary salicylates, as, having ruled out a sulfite sensitivity, it's possible that your asthma is linked to aspirin and related salicylates found in some foods (see pages 48–49). If, after following the full-strength program for one month, your asthma has still not significantly improved, then you may have an idiosyncratic intolerance to some other component of your diet, such as cows' milk proteins, wheat, yeast or eggs. For this reason I'd like you to consult a nutritional therapist who specializes in elimination diets – he or she will be able to identify which individual foods aggravate your asthma (see page 44).

Select the program that's best for you

Instead of following the programs sequentially, another approach is to work out from the start which one is best suited to your needs. You'll need to be able to pinpoint the foods that make your symptoms worse. If you're unsure of the relationship between what you eat and your asthma symptoms, it helps to keep a food-and-symptom diary for at least a week – write down what you eat and when you eat it; also make a note of any wheezing, breathlessness or other respiratory symptoms and the time at which they occur.

Once you've answered the 23 questions on the following two pages you should be ready to select the program that will suit you best.

- If all of your answers are As, start with the gentle program.
- If your answers include one or more Bs, start on the moderate program – your answers suggest dietary sulfites make your asthma worse.
- If you get one or more Cs in your answers, start on the full-strength program – your answers suggest dietary salicylates make your asthma worse.
- If you get some B/Cs in your answers, start with the moderate program first.

1 How often do you eat processed or pre-packaged foods?

- Several times a day   **A**
- Several times a week   **B**
- Hardly ever   **C**

2 How many servings of fruit and vegetables do you eat per day?

- Less than five servings per day   **A**
- Four or five servings per day   **B**
- More than five servings per day   **C**

3 How often do you eat fish?

- Hardly ever   **A**
- Once or twice a week   **B**
- Three or more times a week   **C**

4 How often do you eat take-aways?

- Most days   **A**
- Several times a week   **B**
- Occasionally   **C**

5 Are your asthma symptoms worse after eating dehydrated or dried fruit and vegetables (but not fresh)?

- Don't know   **A**
- Yes   **B**
- No   **A**

6 Are your asthma symptoms worse after eating grapes or drinking grape juice?

- Don't know   **A**
- Yes   **B/C**
- No   **A**

7 Are your asthma symptoms worse after eating fresh ginger?

- Don't know   **A**
- Yes   **C**
- No   **A**

8 Are your asthma symptoms worse after eating dried or preserved ginger?

- Don't know   **A**
- Yes   **B/C**
- No   **A**

9 Are your asthma symptoms worse after eating gherkins?

- Don't know   **A**
- Yes   **B/C**
- No   **A**

10 Are your asthma symptoms worse after drinking wine?

- Don't know   **A**
- Yes   **B/C**
- No   **A**

11 Are your asthma symptoms worse after eating prunes?

- Don't know   **A**
- Yes   **B/C**
- No   **A**

12 Are your asthma symptoms worse after eating tomato paste/ketchup or purée, but not fresh tomatoes?

- Don't know   **A**
- Yes   **B/C**
- No   **A**

13 Are your asthma symptoms worse after eating dried apricots?

- Don't know   A
- Yes   B/C
- No   A

14 Are your asthma symptoms worse after eating canned bamboo shoots?

- Don't know   A
- Yes   B
- No   A

15 Are your asthma symptoms worse after eating pickled or vinegary foods?

- Don't know   A
- Yes   B
- No   A

16 Are your asthma symptoms worse after handling some food-grade plastic bags?

- Don't know   A
- Yes   B
- No   A

17 Are your asthma symptoms worse after eating fresh apricots?

- Don't know   A
- Yes   C
- No   A/B

18 Are your asthma symptoms worse after taking aspirin?

- Don't know   A
- Yes   C
- No   A

19 Are your asthma symptoms worse after taking ibuprofen?

- Don't know   A
- Yes   C
- No   A

20 Are your asthma symptoms worse after eating fresh asparagus?

- Don't know   A
- Yes   C
- No   A

21 Are your asthma symptoms worse after eating a curry?

- Don't know   A
- Yes   C
- No   A

22 Are your asthma symptoms worse after eating licorice?

- Don't know   A
- Yes   C
- No   A

23 Are your asthma symptoms worse after drinking tea?

- Don't know   A
- Yes   C
- No   A

monitoring your progress

Whichever program you decide to follow, it's important to monitor your asthma symptoms closely throughout. If you write them in a diary, this helps you pinpoint the foods that may be making your symptoms worse. The relationship between food and symptoms isn't always clear cut, but in time you may see a pattern.

Another good way to monitor your asthma is to record your peak flow measurements from day to day. Make some copies of the chart below and fill it in every day that you are following a program. As well as peak flow measurements, I've included space for you to record how many puffs of your reliever inhaler you need a day.

Remember – when following any of the programs on the following pages, continue to avoid any foods that you know from experience can trigger your asthma symptoms. Replace these foods with a similar food that you know doesn't trigger your asthma.

Peak flow and puffer diary

Before you start a program, write down your current personal best peak flow reading here: _____

Write down the drugs you are using as part of your asthma management plan here: _____

During a program, measure your peak flow two to four times a day and record it in this chart. Also record how often you need to use your reliever inhaler, and the number of puffs you need to take. Remember, if you need to use your reliever inhaler more than twice a week, you should usually be using a regular preventer inhaler every day, as well.

day	peak flow readings	number of puffs of reliever inhaler
1		
2		
3		
4		
5		
6		
7		

After following a program, your peak flow readings should have improved. Write down your new personal best peak flow reading here: _____ Even if your personal best peak flow reading doesn't improve, your average peak flow reading should.

introducing the gentle program

The gentle program makes following an asthma-friendly diet and lifestyle as easy as possible. Do the program for at least four weeks; you can achieve this by repeating the 14 daily plans that follow.

The gentle program diet

The most important thing I ask you to do in the gentle program diet is to cut back on foods that contain added omega-6 vegetable fats. These promote inflammation in the body and include pre-packaged convenience meals, and snacks such as cakes, biscuits and pastries.

In their place, I ask you to eat more sources of omega-3 fatty acids, such as almonds, walnuts, pumpkin seeds, flax seeds (linseeds) and oily fish. (If you're unable to eat nuts because they trigger your asthma, eat extra seeds instead.)

You'll notice that on the daily menu plans I include fish four times a week, and meat only once or twice a week. Pregnant women or women who are planning to have a baby may want to follow the recommendation in some countries that they restrict oily fish consumption to twice a week (if this applies to you, eat lean meats such as chicken, turkey and lean steak instead). This measure is designed to reduce your exposure to possible pollutants, such as mercury, that are found in deep sea fish and which may have a harmful effect on a developing baby. My recommended supplement plan includes omega-3 fish oil capsules – these are screened for pollutants – so you will still obtain useful amounts of these essential fatty acids, even if you cut back on your fish intake.

The gentle program includes lots of fresh fruit – especially apples, apple juice and bananas – plus a high intake of tomatoes, carrots and fresh green leafy vegetables. Research suggests that these vitamin-mineral- and antioxidant-rich foods can significantly reduce the frequency and severity of asthma attacks, and reduce your need to use inhalers. Other asthma superfoods (see pages 56–59) also feature regularly.

Drink fluids I advise you to drink plenty of fluids on the gentle program – especially mineral water that contains good amounts of calcium and magnesium. Herbal teas, such as camomile, are also beneficial, as are antioxidant-rich black, green and white tea. You don't need to limit coffee or cocoa as these contain ingredients such as caffeine and theobromine that have a bronchodilating action. You may also drink up to 150ml (5¼fl oz) red wine a day, assuming it doesn't worsen your asthma. Select organic wines that have no added sulfites (see pages 46–47).

Foods to avoid or eat less of As well as cutting back on foods containing omega-6 fats, I'd also like you to eliminate table salt from your diet – note that none of the recipes includes salt. Obtain flavour from fresh herbs and black pepper instead. Initially food may taste bland, but over the course of the month you will start to notice how much better fresh, unsalted food can taste. Please don't be tempted to add salt during cooking or at the table, or you will not gain optimum benefits from the gentle program.

Shopping list

These are the items that feature in my suggested menu plans for the next 14 days. Where possible, buy produce regularly for optimum freshness.

drinks
dry white wine, elderberry cordial, fruit tea, green, black or white tea, ground coffee, herbal teas (camomile), mineral water (low sodium), red grape juice, red wine, unsweetened apple juice

dairy products
butter (unsalted), low-fat crème fraîche, low-fat fromage frais (plain and vanilla), mozzarella, Parmesan cheese, plain low-fat bio yogurt, plain low-fat cottage cheese, semi-skimmed/skimmed cows' milk

fruit
apples (dessert and cooking), apricots (fresh and dried), bananas, blackcurrants, blueberries, cherries, clementines, cranberries, grapefruit*, grapes (black, red, green), kumquats, lemons, limes, mangoes, melons, oranges, papaya, peaches, pears, pineapple, plums, pomegranates, raspberries, redcurrants, rhubarb, strawberries. *Check for interactions between grapefruit and your medication

vegetables and salad stuff
avocados, aubergines, broccoli (purple sprouting), carrots, corn on the cob, courgettes, cucumber, dark green cabbage, fennel, green beans, kale, mixed salad leaves, mushrooms (button), onions, peas, potatoes, pumpkin, red cabbage, red, yellow, orange and green peppers, rocket, shallots, spinach, spring greens, spring onions, sweet potatoes, sweetcorn, tomatoes, watercress

nuts and seeds
almonds, Brazils, flax seeds (linseeds), pine nuts, pumpkin seeds, sunflower seeds, walnuts

herbs and spices
basil, black pepper, bay leaf, chives, chillies, cinnamon, coriander leaf, coriander seeds, dill, garlic, mint, oregano, parsley, rosemary, tarragon, thyme (lemon and garden)

oils, vinegars and condiments
balsamic vinegar, extra virgin olive oil (for drizzling and dressings), olive oil (for cooking), red wine vinegar, walnut oil, wholegrain mustard

grains
bread rolls, breakfast cereals (high-fibre cereals, rolled porridge oats, wheatgerm, wholewheat), brown rice, couscous, pitta bread, plain flour, red rice, wholegrain bread, wholemeal pasta (conchiglie, fettuccine, spaghetti), wholewheat flour

proteins
adzuki beans, anchovies, butter beans, broad beans, chicken, cod, kidney beans, lamb, mackerel, omega-3-enriched eggs, prawns, salmon, sardines, sole, trout

miscellaneous
brandy, brown sugar, caster sugar, cornflour, dark chocolate (at least 70 percent cocoa solids), filo pastry, fish stock, Grand Marnier or Cointreau, honey, soy sauce, tomato purée, vegetable bouillon, Worcestershire sauce

Losing weight Although the gentle program is not specifically designed to help you lose weight, you may find that you lose any excess weight slowly and naturally. This is because you are eating healthily and avoiding high intakes of refined carbohydrates and dietary fats. Losing excess weight can reduce the level of inflammation in your body and alleviate your asthma symptoms. If you want to accelerate the process of weight loss, eat smaller portions than those I suggest in the program, and omit or eat smaller amounts of the starchy foods on your menu, such as wholemeal toast, rolls, pasta, rice and couscous.

The gentle program breathing exercises

Many people with asthma hold their upper chest and shoulders in a position of partial inhalation – this overworks the respiratory muscles and requires a lot more energy than normal. As part of the gentle program, I show you a series of exercises that can help to relax your upper body, and improve your respiratory function and asthma control. The exercises may even reduce your need for reliever inhalers. In one study, carried out in Australia, breathing techniques and upper-body exercises helped the 57 participants reduce their use of inhalers by 86 percent and to step down the use of their preventer inhaler by 50 percent within 12 weeks. At the start of the study, reliever inhalers were used an average of three puffs a day. After one month of doing breathing exercises twice a day, reliever-inhaler use fell to an average of one puff every three days. Instead of reaching for their inhalers, the participants had started to use breathing exercises to regain breath control. They used two different types of exercise: one focused on shallow nasal breathing, shallow breathing and breath-holding; the other focused on non-specific upper-body exercises with no attempt to change the pattern of breathing. The benefits of both programs were the same.

Gentle program supplements

I suggest you take the following supplements during the gentle program. Those in the recommended list are likely to have a beneficial effect on your asthma symptoms. Those in the optional list have the potential to alleviate your symptoms even further. See pages 60–61 for a discussion of these supplements.

recommended daily supplements

- Vitamin C (500mg)
- Vitamin E (200mg)
- B-vitamin complex (25mg)
- Lycopene carotenoid complex (15mg)
- Magnesium (300mg)
- Selenium (50mcg)
- Omega-3 fish oils (1g fish oil capsules, each supplying 180mg EPA + 120mg DHA)
- Pycnogenol (50mg)

optional daily supplements (these provide additional benefits)

- Co-enzyme Q10 (30mg)
- Quercetin (500mg, three times a day before food)
- N-acetyl-l-cysteine (NAC) (100mg, three times a day)
- Reishi (500mg)
- Digestive enzymes (mixed; 1 capsule before meals)
- Green-lipped mussel extracts (350mg, three times a day)
- Folic acid (400mcg) plus vitamin B12 (50mcg)
- Probiotics (in the form of fermented milk drinks, bio yogurt or supplements)

Throughout the gentle program I show you similar exercises to improve your breathing. Whenever you feel your asthma symptoms starting, try using these exercises for relief. However, if shortness of breath or wheeziness persist, it's important to use your inhaler according to your personal asthma management plan.

Aerobic exercise As well as doing the daily breathing exercises, I'd like you to exercise for at least 15 minutes per day at a rate that is brisk enough to raise your pulse rate about 100 beats per minute and to leave you feeling slightly breathless. Over the course of the month, gradually build up in time and intensity until you achieve 30 minutes brisk exercise on at least five days per week to improve your general cardiorespiratory health. Brisk walking is one of the easiest ways to achieve and maintain fitness, and is least likely to affect your asthma. Note: you don't have to do 30 minutes of exercise all in one go – you can do three sessions of 10 minutes each if you prefer.

If you have problems with exercise-induced asthma, follow the advice on pages 68–69 and use your reliever inhaler 15 minutes before starting to exercise.

The gentle program therapies

During the first week I show you how essential oils can help you relax and improve your breathing. During the second week, I introduce a number of different complementary approaches so you can evaluate which you find most helpful. Please book an appointment with an aromatherapist and a homeopath (see pages 174 and 175) before you start the program.

the gentle program day one

Daily menu

- **Breakfast: Full-of-Goodness Cereal (see page 100) with blueberries**

- **Morning snack: a large apple**

- **Lunch: Home-made Tomato Soup (see page 88). Brown roll. Bowl of mixed salad leaves drizzled with walnut oil and lemon juice and sprinkled with flax seeds (linseeds). Low-fat bio yogurt with fresh fruit**

- **Afternoon snack: a small banana**

- **Dinner: Creamy Salmon in Filo Parcels (see page 104). Spinach. Baked cherry tomatoes. New potatoes. Handful of black grapes**

- **Drinks: semi-skimmed or skimmed milk. Three or four cups of ground coffee or cocoa. Apple or red grape juice. Elderberry cordial. Unlimited green/black/white tea, camomile tea and mineral water**

- **Supplements: see page 81**

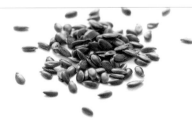

Daily breathing exercise

Over the next two weeks, I'm going to show you some simple exercises. Do these once in the morning and once in the evening. Today's exercise involves a simple relaxing breath – do it to classical music if you like. Once you've mastered the technique, use this slow, gentle form of breathing all the time in your everyday life.

Relaxing breath

1 Sit comfortably. Imagine a string attached to the top of your head pulling you up straight as your upper body relaxes. Don't tense your shoulders.

2 Breathe in slowly and gently through your nose, and out through your mouth. Relax into the breath so the air expels itself – rather than being forced out by your muscles. Aim to spend around twice as long exhaling as you do inhaling. Do this for at least five minutes.

Aromatherapy

Essential oils with anti-spasmodic, anti-allergy, anti-inflammatory and decongestant properties can all help your breathing. Over the next week I'll show you how to use selected oils. Today I suggest you start with lavender essential oil, which suits most people. When you go to bed tonight, place four drops of pure, natural lavender essential oil on a tissue and tuck it under your pillow. You can also put some drops on a piece of cottonwool and place it in a locket or small vial to sniff during the day.

Wear medical ID

!

When you have asthma it's a good idea to wear a bracelet, watch or pendant (or carry a key fob) that records information about your condition. The MedicAlert range of products are recognized worldwide and provide important information needed by doctors and paramedics in an emergency. They are engraved with your personal ID number and medical facts, such as your medication. This is especially important if you use oral steroids.

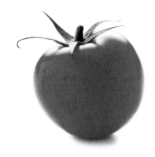

day two

Daily menu

- **Breakfast: bowl of high-fibre cereal sprinkled with almonds, raspberries and flax seeds (linseeds)**

- **Morning snack: a large apple**

- **Lunch: Anchovy and Red Pepper Spread (see page 101). Wholegrain toast. Fruit, for example, a bowl of cherries**

- **Afternoon snack: a small banana**

- **Dinner: Spaghetti with Tomato and Mozzarella Cheese (see instructions opposite). Fruit Crumble (see page 108)**

- **Drinks: semi-skimmed or skimmed milk. Three or four cups of ground coffee or cocoa. Apple or red grape juice. Elderberry cordial. Unlimited green/black/white tea, camomile tea and mineral water**

- **Supplements: see page 81**

If your asthma is triggered by exercise, it's a good idea to eat lots of tomatoes. They contain lycopene, which can help prevent an attack. Today's dinner is a simple but delicious way to use fresh tomatoes – simply heat the chopped flesh in a pan with some olive oil, crushed garlic, mozzarella cheese and oregano, then toss with hot spaghetti and sprinkle with Parmesan.

Daily breathing exercise

Today, I'm going to show you an exercise used by opera singers – it's great for clearing your nostrils.

Nostril-clearing breath

1 Sit with your mouth closed. Breathe in through both nostrils as normal, then close your right nostril by placing your right thumb against it. Breathe out through your left nostril, then close your left nostril by pushing your right index finger against it. At the same time, release your thumb so your right nostril opens. Breathe in through your right nostril.

2 Close your right nostril and breathe out through the left nostril. Repeat 10 times, then reverse the order (closing your nostrils with your left thumb and index finger), so you breathe in through the left nostril and out through the right.

3 Return to yesterday's relaxing breath – in through your nose and out through your mouth. Notice how clear your nostrils feel. Practise both exercises whenever your nostrils feel blocked.

Aromatherapy

Today's therapeutic technique is an anti-spasmodic aromatherapy bath before you go to bed. Add the following essential oils to 15ml carrier oil (see page 25): two drops each of camomile, lavender and neroli. Draw your bath so that it is comfortably warm, then add the oil mixture once the taps are turned off. Keep the lights low and soak for 15 minutes with your eyes closed. You should feel comfortable and relaxed afterwards, so take the opportunity to go straight to bed and enjoy a good night's sleep. Use lavender oil under your pillow again tonight.

the gentle program day three

Daily menu

- **Breakfast: smoothie made by whizzing mango, papaya and blackcurrants in a food processor**

- **Morning snack: a large apple**

- **Lunch: bowl of cottage cheese mixed with chopped pineapple, and pomegranate. Wholegrain roll. Handful of walnuts**

- **Afternoon snack: a small banana**

- **Dinner: Coq au Vin Rouge (see page 106). Red rice. Broccoli. Carrots. Mixed berries with fromage frais**

- **Drink suggestions: semi-skimmed or skimmed milk. Three or four cups of ground coffee or cocoa. Apple or red grape juice. Elderberry cordial. Unlimited green/black/white tea, camomile tea and mineral water**

- **Supplements: see page 81**

Daily breathing exercise

Today, I want you to focus on diaphragmatic breathing – using your diaphragm to draw air into your lungs.

Diaphragmatic breathing

1 Sit, stand or lie with your feet apart while resting your hands lightly on your abdomen. Breathe in through your nose and out through your mouth. Note whether your shoulders and chest rise and fall, or your abdomen rises and falls.

2 If you notice most of the movement in your shoulders and chest, make a conscious effort to draw air down into your belly using your diaphragm. Keep your shoulders and chest still. Feel your abdomen rise and fall as you breathe in and out.

Aromatherapy

Camomile has soothing, calming, anti-spasmodic, anti-allergy and anti-inflammatory properties. German camomile has a stronger action than Roman camomile as it contains greater quantities of anti-inflammatory chamazulene.

This substance, which isn't present in the plant itself, is produced by chemical reactions during distillation, and gives the oil a beautiful blue colour. Put two drops of German camomile essential oil on some cottonwool and place in a small plastic box or stoppered glass vial. Open and inhale the scent regularly throughout the day. Drink camomile tea for its soothing, stress-relieving properties.

Play a wind instrument

Taking up a wind instrument, such as the flute, clarinet or oboe, can significantly improve asthma symptoms by teaching you breath control, strengthening your respiratory muscles and improving your lung capacity. In a study of teenagers with asthma, those who played a wind instrument experienced fewer asthma symptoms, panic attacks and mood changes, and less fatigue than those who didn't. They also felt better able to cope with their asthma.

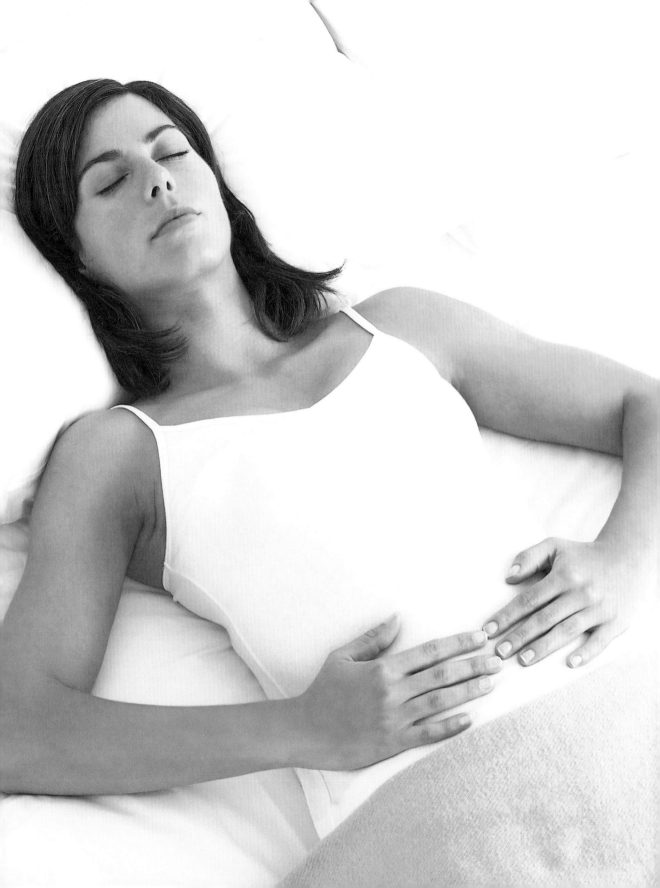

the gentle program day four

Daily menu

- Breakfast: Wholewheat, Nuts and Blueberries (see page 100)

- Morning snack: a large apple

- Lunch: bowl of mixed beans and chopped tomatoes sprinkled with grated carrot, walnuts and pumpkin seeds. Wholegrain roll. Low-fat bio yogurt with fresh fruit

- Afternoon snack: a small banana

- Dinner: Mackerel with Mustard and Herbs (see page 106). Baked potato. Courgettes. Sweetcorn. 40–50g (about 1½oz) bar dark chocolate (70 percent cocoa solids)

- Drinks: semi-skimmed or skimmed milk. Three or four cups of ground coffee or cocoa. Apple or red grape juice. Elderberry cordial. Unlimited green/black/white tea, camomile tea and mineral water

- Supplements: see page 81

Daily breathing exercise

Here's another exercise used by opera singers – it improves diaphragmatic breath control.

Seated forward bend

1 Sit in a comfortable chair, and lean forward until your stomach touches your upper thighs. Let your arms hang by the sides of your legs – they may reach the floor depending on the height of your chair.

2 Now breathe in slowly and deeply using your diaphragm, so your stomach expands and your upper body moves upward slightly. Then slowly exhale and let your upper body move back down. Don't use your back muscles to move your body up and down – the air entering your lungs and pushing your abdomen in and out is the only force you need.

3 Repeat this 10 times, twice a day from now on.

Avoid cold foods

If your asthma symptoms are brought on by the cold, avoid eating ice cream or drinking extremely cold liquids, such as chilled white wine, ice-laden drinks or frozen cocktails. In some people, exposure to cold foods and drinks shocks the airways into spasm. Some people develop a headache after eating very cold ice cream, too.

Aromatherapy

Rub an essential oil blend into your chest before you go to bed – use the chest rub from page 25. Continue to use lavender essential oil at night to promote sleep. Instead of using cottonwool, you could buy a lavender pillow or posy containing dried lavender flowers.

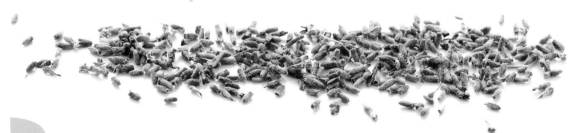

day five

Daily menu

- **Breakfast: Full-of-Goodness Cereal (see page 100) with cherries**

- **Morning snack: a large apple**

- **Lunch: Prawn and Papaya Citrus Salad (see page 102). Wholegrain roll. Handful of Brazil nuts**

- **Afternoon snack: a small banana**

- **Dinner: Aubergines Parmesan (see page 104). Kale. Green beans. Tangy Apple Swirl (see page 108)**

- **Drinks: semi-skimmed or skimmed milk. Three or four cups of ground coffee or cocoa. Apple or red grape juice. Elderberry cordial. Unlimited green/black/white tea, camomile tea and mineral water**

- **Supplements: see page 81**

Elderberry cordial appears every day in my drink suggestions on the gentle program. Elderberries contain a number of powerful antioxidant pigments, known as anthocyanins, which help to dry up catarrh and reduce inflammation in the respiratory tract, whether you have hayfever or a viral infection. They're particularly effective against viral infections and, in my experience, can stop a cold in its tracks within 24 hours. Eat elderberry jam, drink elderberry fruit wine or cordial, or take elderberry supplements.

Daily breathing exercise

Today's exercise helps to strengthen your diaphragm even further.

Diaphragm strengthener

1 Lie on the floor with a pillow under your head. Put a large book on your belly and make it move up and down as you breathe using your diaphragm.
2 When you can do this easily, add another large book and push it upward, as far as you can, using just the power of diaphragmatic breath control.
3 To strengthen your diaphragm further, keep increasing the load. Do the exercise every day for at least five minutes.

Aromatherapy

Marjoram is one of the best essential oils for reducing respiratory spasm and congestion. Put two drops of marjoram essential oil on a piece of cottonwool and place it in a small plastic box or stoppered glass vial. Inhale the scent whenever you produce excess mucus or feel bunged up (don't do this if you're driving or operating machinery as marjoram is also sedative). Alternatively, mix six drops marjoram with 15ml carrier oil and add to a hot bath before bed.

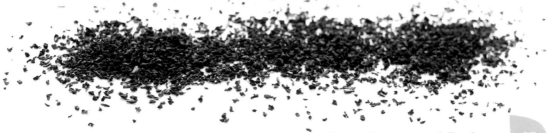

the gentle program
day six

Daily menu

- **Breakfast: a slice of watermelon. Wholegrain toast. Scrambled eggs made with omega-3 enriched eggs**

- **Morning snack: a large apple**

- **Lunch: Home-made Tomato Soup (see box). Brown roll. Bowl of mixed salad leaves drizzled with walnut oil and lemon juice and sprinkled with flax seeds (linseeds). A piece of fruit, for example, a pear**

- **Afternoon snack: a small banana**

- **Dinner: Baked Orange and Rosemary Trout (see page 105). Wholegrain pasta shells. Purple sprouting broccoli. Carrots. Vanilla fromage frais with fresh fruit**

- **Drinks: semi-skimmed or skimmed milk. Three or four cups of ground coffee or cocoa. Apple or red grape juice. Elderberry cordial. Unlimited green/black/white tea, camomile tea and mineral water**

- **Supplements: see page 81**

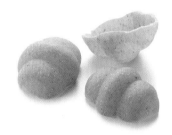

Daily breathing exercise

Today, I show you a deceptively simple exercise called the vacuum – it's excellent for toning and strengthening your abdominal muscles so that diaphragmatic breathing (see day three) becomes easier.

The vacuum

1 To do the vacuum, suck in your stomach as if you're trying to touch your spine with your navel. Draw in your abdomen as far as you can and hold it in for a count of 10.

2 Do this twice a day from now on. With time, try to hold in your abdomen for longer and longer. You don't have to hold your breath while doing this, but you will need to breathe using your chest muscles – usually a no-no – while sucking in your abdomen.

Aromatherapy

When you use an essential oil regularly, it becomes less effective as your body adapts to its therapeutic action. So, instead of lavender oil to promote sleep, start using two drops each of melissa and neroli essential oils near your pillow at night. From now on, I suggest you change your nightly essential oil at least once a week – base your choice on the properties of different essential oils (see page 25), and create blends that you particularly like.

Home-made tomato soup

Make home-made soup a regular part of your diet. To make today's lunchtime soup, sprinkle some tomatoes with chopped garlic and Italian herbs before drizzling them with olive oil and roasting them in the oven for 30–45 minutes. Purée the cooked tomatoes in a blender and dilute with milk or stock. Reheat the soup and season with black pepper and sprinkle herbs on top.

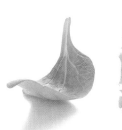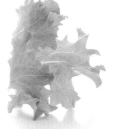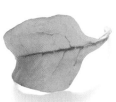

① ② ③ ④ ⑤ ⑥ ⑦

day seven

Daily menu

- Breakfast: Mango Oat-so Smoothie (see page 101)

- Morning snack: piece of fruit

- Lunch: corn on the cob. Bowl of mixed salad leaves drizzled with walnut oil and lemon juice and sprinkled with pumpkin seeds. Wholegrain roll. Low-fat bio yogurt with fresh fruit

- Afternoon snack: a small banana

- Dinner: baby aubergines, courgettes, red onions, tomatoes and peppers sprinkled with chopped garlic and fresh herbs, drizzled with olive oil and roasted until soft. Couscous. Spring greens. Oranges in Caramel (see page 109)

- Drinks: semi-skimmed or skimmed milk. Three or four cups of ground coffee or cocoa. Apple or red grape juice. Elderberry cordial. Unlimited green/black/white tea, camomile tea and mineral water

- Supplements: see page 81

Daily breathing exercise

Today's exercise involves sitting quietly and slowing down your breath.

Slow breathing

1   Sit quietly in a chair. Keep a clock or watch in view. Breathe in through your nose, and out through your mouth (using your diaphragm; see page 84) and count how many breaths you take during the course of a minute. Use your fingers to count if it helps. The average number of breaths per minute by an adult at rest is 12.

2   Slowly reduce your breathing rate – aim for 10 breaths a minute. Make each breath slow and smooth rather than ragged or uneven. Don't gulp air or let it out suddenly.

3   Practise slow breathing for 15 minutes a day, and try to adopt this method of breathing all the time in your everyday life. Slow, gentle breathing helps to relieve stress and anxiety, lower your blood pressure, improve lung efficiency and prevent hyperventilation.

Consulting an aromatherapist

Having followed the gentle program for one week, it's time to consult a complementary therapist for some individual, professional advice. I suggest you have a relaxing yet therapeutic aromatherapy massage. An aromatherapist will select essential oils that improve respiratory function; he or she will massage these diluted oils into your skin for optimum therapeutic effect. Read more about aromatherapy on page 25 and, to find an aromatherapist, go to page 174.

Green tea

Green tea contains powerful antioxidants, known as catechins. They have a natural antihistamine effect and help to maintain a healthy immune system. Drinking two or three cups of green tea daily, especially during the hayfever season, may help to reduce asthma symptoms. Green tea extracts are also available as supplements.

the gentle program day eight

Daily menu

- **Breakfast: smoothie made by whizzing papaya, blueberries and freshly squeezed orange juice in a food processor**

- **Morning snack: a large apple**

- **Lunch: Watercress, Pear and Pomegranate Salad (see page 102). Brown roll. Handful of red grapes**

- **Afternoon snack: a small banana**

- **Dinner: Herby Orange Chicken (see page 106). Brown rice. Peas. Rocket sprinkled with olive oil and balsamic vinegar. 40–50g (about 1½oz) bar dark chocolate (70 percent cocoa solids)**

- **Drinks: semi-skimmed or skimmed milk. Three or four cups of ground coffee or cocoa. Apple or red grape juice. Elderberry cordial. Unlimited green/black/white tea, camomile tea and mineral water**

- **Supplements: see page 81**

Over the next few days I introduce several different complementary therapies that can help people with asthma. Everyone is different, with different needs, likes and dislikes – some approaches will appeal to you, while others may suit you less. Once you've found a therapy that resonates with you, you can research other ways to introduce it into your daily life.

Daily breathing exercise

Today's exercise is the first in a series of four that synchronize breath and movement. This first exercise helps to limber up your chest, shoulder and abdominal muscles, which has been shown to alleviate asthma symptoms and reduce inhaler usage.

Breath and movement 1

1　Stand straight with your feet comfortably apart. As you breathe in gently through your nose using your diaphragm, slowly lift both arms up to meet above your head. Allow your chest to fully expand with air.

2　Slowly bring your arms back down and exhale effortlessly through your mouth in synchrony with the movement. Repeat four more times. Do this twice a day from now on. Work up to 10 or more repetitions.

Hand reflexology

The first complementary technique to try is hand – rather than foot – reflexology, as this is easier to do in public. Whenever your chest starts to feel tight, gently massage the "lung" area, which is located at the base of your middle three fingers, on the palm side of both hands. Massage this area for two minutes on each hand. You can also use the more intensive foot reflexology session I describe on page 33.

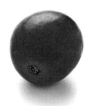

day nine

Daily menu

- **Breakfast: Full-of-Goodness Cereal (see page 100) with blueberries**

- **Morning snack: a large apple**

- **Lunch: home-made vegetable soup, such as mushroom, garlic and fennel (see page 112). Wholegrain roll. Handful of walnuts**

- **Afternoon snack: a small banana**

- **Dinner: Cod in Green Sauce (see page 105). Dark green cabbage. Carrots. Sweet potatoes. Fresh raspberries with vanilla fromage frais**

- **Drinks: semi-skimmed or skimmed milk. Three or four cups of ground coffee or cocoa. Apple or red grape juice. Elderberry cordial. Unlimited green/black/white tea, camomile tea and mineral water**

- **Supplements: see page 81**

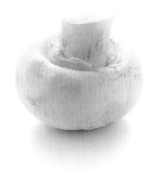

Daily breathing exercise

Today you're going to repeat the breath and movement exercise you learned yesterday, but as you breathe out I want you to make a sound.

Breath and movement 2

1 Stand straight with your feet comfortably apart. As you breathe in gently through your nose using your diaphragm, slowly lift both arms up to meet above your head. Allow your chest to fully expand with air.

2 Squeeze your buttock muscles tightly together and stretch backward slightly as you release all the air from your mouth and make a long "aaahhhhh" sound. Let the tension flow out of you.

3 When you've finished exhaling, release any remaining tension by moving your upper body in small circular movements.

4 Stand up straight, lower your arms and repeat the previous steps four times. Do this exercise twice a day from now on. Build up to 10 or more repetitions.

Onion marmalade

Onions are a rich dietary source of quercetin and have a powerful antihistamine action. Try making onion marmalade to accompany meat, fish, vegetable or cheese dishes. Simply peel and chop four large onions and stir-fry in a pan with olive oil until well-coated. Cover and leave to sweat and caramelize on low heat for 30 minutes. Remove the lid and cook for a further 10 minutes to reduce excess moisture. Serve hot.

Homeopathy

Although it's best to consult a homeopath for individual advice, there are some remedies you can try by yourself. Look at the chart on page 30 and select the remedy that most accurately describes your situation. For example, if you have exercise-induced asthma, *Ambra grisea* is likely to suit you. Buy a vial of your chosen remedy at the 6c dilution, and take it twice a day for five days. Follow the guidelines on page 29.

the gentle program day ten

Daily menu

- **Breakfast: Minty Mango and Melon Medley (see page 101)**

- **Morning snack: a large apple**

- **Lunch: sliced avocado with pomegranate seeds. Bowl of mixed salad leaves drizzled with walnut oil and lemon juice and sprinkled with flax seeds (linseeds). Fromage frais with fresh fruit**

- **Afternoon snack: a small banana**

- **Dinner: Creamy Salmon in Filo Parcels (see page 104). Bowl of mixed salad leaves, tomato and red onion slices sprinkled with olive oil and balsamic vinegar. Strawberries in fresh orange juice**

- **Drinks: semi-skimmed or skimmed milk. Three or four cups of ground coffee or cocoa. Apple or red grape juice. Elderberry cordial. Unlimited green/black/white tea, camomile tea and mineral water**

- **Supplements: see page 81**

Daily breathing exercise

Repeat the exercises from days eight and nine, then add the following exercise.

Breath and movement 3

1 Stand comfortably, with your feet apart and your arms by your sides. As you breathe in through your nostrils (using your diaphragm), slowly lift both arms out to the sides, palms downward, until they are parallel to the ground.

2 Hold this position for one second, then breathe out slowly through your mouth as you lower your arms. Repeat 10 times. For maximum benefit, do this exercise while holding weights (cans of food are fine).

Herbalism

I'd like you to start using a herbal medicine to help your asthma symptoms. The one I've selected for the gentle program is curcumin

Flower remedies

Anxiety can trigger an asthma attack so it's important to learn ways to manage anxious, panicky feelings. Try using a flower remedy (this is a homeopathic flower essence preserved in brandy). Add five drops of Rescue Remedy or Australian Bush Flower Emergency Essence to a glass of water and sip slowly, every three to five minutes, holding the liquid in your mouth for a while. Alternatively, place five drops directly on your tongue.

– an anti-inflammatory extract from the yellow curry spice turmeric. Take a 400mg supplement twice a day. If you prefer to take curcumin in the traditional Ayurvedic way, simply mix a teaspoon of fresh turmeric powder in a glass of milk. Drink it on an empty stomach twice a day.

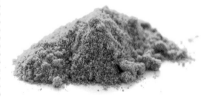
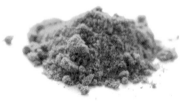

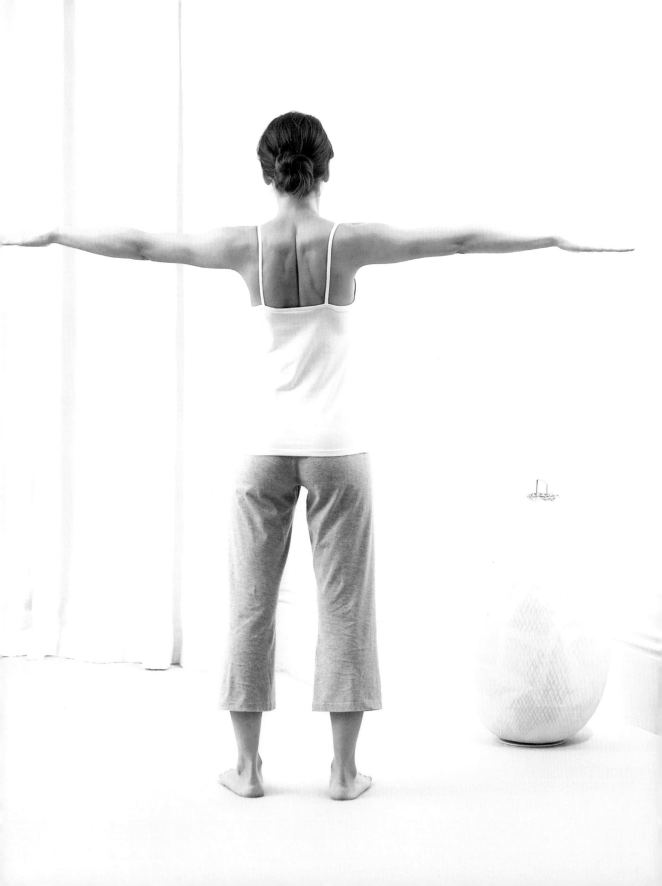

the gentle program
day eleven

Daily menu

- **Breakfast: bowl of high-fibre cereal sprinkled with almonds, flax seeds (linseeds) and pomegranate seeds**

- **Morning snack: a large apple**

- **Lunch: Baked Peppers with Tomato Stuffing (see page 102). Wholegrain roll. A handful of Brazil nuts**

- **Afternoon snack: a small banana**

- **Dinner: Lamb alla Romana (see page 106). Brown rice. Spinach. Carrots. Baked tomatoes. A handful of cherries**

- **Drinks: semi-skimmed or skimmed milk. Three or four cups of ground coffee or cocoa. Apple or red grape juice. Elderberry cordial. Unlimited green/black/white tea, camomile tea and mineral water**

- **Supplements: see page 81**

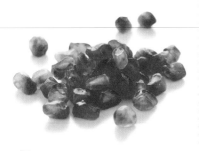

Dehydration stimulates histamine release in the airways, so remember to drink plenty of water each day. Keep a bottle of mineral water (also a good source of magnesium) with you at all times and sip it regularly throughout the day. Your thirst receptors are not very efficient – by the time you feel thirsty you are already significantly dehydrated, so prevention is the best ploy. Drink extra water when drinking caffeinated drinks or alcohol, as these have a diuretic action.

Daily breathing exercise

Repeat the exercises from days eight to 10 and then add the final exercise of the series.

Breath and movement 4

1   Stand comfortably with your feet apart and your arms by your sides. As you take a slow breath through your nostrils (using your diaphragm), lift both arms out in front of you until they are parallel to the ground. Rotate your palms so they face the ceiling.

2   Hold this position for one second, then breathe out

slowly as you lower your arms back down. Repeat 10 times. For maximum benefit, do this exercise while holding weights (or food cans).

Acupressure

Stimulating a point known as Lung 5, or Foot Marsh, is beneficial for people with asthma – see below. Other useful points are Stomach 16, Lung 1 and Urinary Bladder 13 (see box on page 36).

Stimulating Lung 5

1   The lung meridian runs along the arm where there is a visible change in your skin colour and texture. Feel down this line, from your arm crease, until you find a point that feels tender on your inner forearm, just below the crease of your elbow on the thumb side of your arm.

2   Press this acupoint for 10 seconds. Relax and repeat. Do the same on your other arm. Do this often to strengthen your lungs. If you cannot find an obviously tender point, press 2.5cm (1in) away from your elbow crease on the lung meridian.

day twelve

Daily menu

- Breakfast: watermelon slice. Wholegrain toast. Boiled omega-3-enriched egg

- Morning snack: a large apple

- Lunch: grilled tomatoes on wholegrain toast. Bowl of mixed salad leaves drizzled with walnut oil and lemon juice and sprinkled with pumpkin seeds. A piece of fruit, for example, a peach

- Afternoon snack: a small banana

- Dinner: Sole with Red Wine and Grapes (see page 105). Mashed pumpkin. Broccoli. 40–50g (about 1½oz) bar dark chocolate (70 percent cocoa solids)

- Drinks: semi-skimmed or skimmed milk. Three or four cups of ground coffee or cocoa. Apple or red grape juice. Elderberry cordial. Unlimited green/black/white tea, camomile tea and mineral water

- Supplements: see page 81

Daily breathing exercise

This exercise, known as "huffing", helps to clear excess mucus from your lungs.

Huffing

1 Breathe in, then sharply tighten your abdominal muscles to push the air out as quickly as you can using your stomach muscles only – imagine you are blowing out candles on a cake.

2 Aim to make a huffing sound. If your exhalations sound more like whooshes, you're using your chest muscles as well as your abdominals. Try again until you make a huff.

3 Do as many huffs as you can to help clear mucus from your lungs – with practice you'll build up the stamina to do 20 or more. This will bring mucus to the top of your airways so you can clear it with a cough. Repeat several times a day, as often as you need to.

Meditation

Try this simple meditation technique – it helps to reduce the frequency of stress-related asthma attacks.

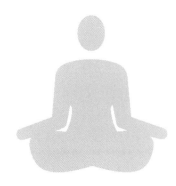

Colour meditation

1 Sit comfortably in a chair with your eyes shut. Picture the healing dark blue colour of indigo. Imagine the colour swirling behind your eyelids in a moving cloud.

2 Let your body relax and try to fill your imagination with indigo. The more colour you can visualize, the stronger the healing effect. If your mind wanders, just keep returning to focus on the colour.

3 When you feel ready, bring your mind slowly back, open your eyes and enjoy the sense of calm that flows through you. Try to meditate for at least five minutes once a day, initially, building up to 15 or more minutes as you find it easier to let go.

the gentle program
day thirteen

Daily menu

- **Breakfast: Sardine Fishcakes (see page 100)**

- **Morning snack: a large apple**

- **Lunch: bowl of chopped pear, walnuts and cottage cheese. Wholegrain roll. Low-fat bio yogurt with blueberries**

- **Afternoon snack: a small banana**

- **Dinner: fettuccine sprinkled with pine nuts, walnuts, grated Parmesan, chopped parsley and oregano and drizzled with garlic-infused olive oil. Tomato, sliced red onion and rocket leaves drizzled with olive oil and balsamic vinegar. Bittersweet Fruit Compote (see page 108)**

- **Drinks: semi-skimmed or skimmed milk. Three or four cups of ground coffee or cocoa. Apple or red grape juice. Elderberry cordial. Unlimited green/black/white tea, camomile tea and mineral water**

- **Supplements: see page 81**

Daily breathing exercise

Like yesterday's huffing exercise, pursing helps you to bring up excess mucus so that you can cough it out. Do it straight after huffing (see day twelve).

Pursing

1 Breathe in, then sharply tighten your abdominal muscles to push the air out as quickly as you can through your pursed lips. Make a series of tiny, forceful "pffff" sounds.

2 Clear the mucus that comes to the top of your airways with a cough. Repeat several times a day, as often as you need to.

Air purification

A good natural approach to treating asthma is to use a negative ionizer (see page 63). Start looking into buying one today. Ionizers effectively remove airborne particles, such as pollen and dust from your indoor atmosphere. They also have a calming effect by neutralizing stress-inducing positive ions from the air. Some ionizers have an integral aromatherapy facility to scent the air with essential oils, too. The most natural negative ionizer is a rock salt crystal lamp in which a lump of ancient rock salt is hollowed out to hold a candle. The resulting atmosphere allows you to enjoy a little speleotherapy in your own home (see page 62). Himalayan and Polish rock salt crystal lamps are peach-pink in colour; Persian lamps are white, or lavender and white.

Moving on to the moderate program

You have now completed a substantial part of the gentle program. If your symptoms have improved and you decide to stay on the gentle program in the long term, that's great. However, I recommend that you also try the breathing exercises in the moderate program. They are based on the Buteyko method of breathing, which may improve asthma symptoms to the point where you become even less dependent on your asthma inhalers.

day fourteen

Daily menu

- **Breakfast: Full-of-Goodness Cereal (see page 100) with blueberries**

- **Morning snack: a large apple**

- **Lunch: Gazpacho (see page 101). Wholegrain roll. Fromage frais with fresh fruit**

- **Afternoon snack: a small banana**

- **Dinner: salmon steak sprinkled with chopped garlic and herbs, then grilled. Sweetcorn. Spring greens. Pears in Citrus Red Wine (see page 108)**

- **Drinks: semi-skimmed or skimmed milk. Three or four cups of ground coffee or cocoa. Apple or red grape juice. Elderberry cordial. Unlimited green/black/white tea, camomile tea and mineral water**

- **Supplements: see page 81**

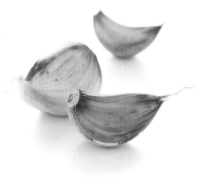

In future, whenever you feel an asthma attack coming on, focus on breathing out rather than breathing in, even though this goes against your instincts when you are feeling breathless. Use your diaphragm, as well as your chest muscles to help push air out of your lungs. Breathing out fully not only calms you but creates more space for fresh air to enter your lungs.

Daily breathing exercise

Do the huffing and pursing exercises that you learned on days twelve and thirteen.

Consulting a homeopath

Having followed the gentle program for two weeks you should have noticed a significant improvement in your asthma symptoms. It's now time to think about consulting another practitioner, and I suggest you see a homeopath. You selected a homeopathic remedy on day nine, which you have taken for the last five days. A homeopath will be able to assess whether you would benefit from a different remedy based not just on your symptoms but on your constitutional type.

> **Stress diary**
> Keep a stress diary, and try to work out which situations or people make you feel stressed enough to bring on your asthma. Try to avoid these situations. If they are unavoidable, talk to your doctor about using your reliever inhaler before a stressful encounter.

Homeopaths recognize 15 different constitutional types, based on factors such as your build, personality, likes, dislikes and emotions. Prescribing according to your constitutional type is particularly important when treating a long-term condition such as asthma, for which several different treatment options are available.

A homeopath will ask you a series of detailed questions before prescribing a remedy. You will also have a follow-up appointment in a few weeks' time to review your response to treatment. To find a homeopath, check the resources at the end of this book.

continuing the gentle program

Congratulations – you have now followed the gentle program for two weeks. I suggest you repeat the eating plan one more time to extend the program to one month. This will give you a good understanding of the dietary changes you need to make. After this, feel free to make your own adjustments to take into account your own likes, dislikes and lifestyle – as well as continuing to exclude any foods you have identified as triggering your asthma symptoms. Start varying the foods you eat, and include new recipes for variety. You will find some suggestions at www.naturalhealthguru.co.uk and you can post your own favourite recipes for other followers of the program to try. If the gentle program works for you, and your asthma symptoms are well controlled, aim to follow its principles for the rest of your life.

Your long-term diet
Essentially, the gentle program diet is a healthy way to eat that includes lots of fresh fruit and vegetables, plus selected nuts and oily fish for their high omega-3 essential fatty acid content. When eating hen's eggs, select omega-3-enriched versions. When eating oily fish, choose any from this list: anchovies, bloater, cacha, carp, eel, herring, hilsa, jack fish, katla, kipper, mackerel, orange roughy, pangas, pilchards, salmon, sardines, sprats, swordfish, trout, tuna (fresh, not canned) and whitebait.

Continue to eat wholegrain bread, pasta and cereals rather than processed white versions, and continue to exclude processed, pre-packaged foods that tend to contain high amounts of the omega-6 essential fatty acids – these are converted into inflammatory substances in the body. If you need to lose weight, or if you're inactive, cut back on the amount of carbohydrate you eat, and try to increase the amount of exercise you take. Aim to eat only as much as you need to feel full. Don't feel you have to finish everything on your plate – you can always eat a bit more in an hour or two if you feel hungry again. In fact, having several small meals a day is more beneficial for weight loss than eating larger meals three times a day.

Concentrate on eating at least four or five servings of salad stuff and vegetables (not including potatoes) and two or three servings of fruit per day as

What if healthy foods trigger my asthma attacks?
If you recognize that certain foods trigger your asthma symptoms, cut them out of your diet even if they are a recognized asthma superfood. Everyone is different and your immune system may have developed an oversensitivity to certain foods. Consulting a naturopath or a nutritionist with training in the field of food intolerances will help you to pinpoint which foods you react against. A naturopath or nutritionist will also be able to tell you how to eat a healthy and balanced diet while avoiding your trigger foods.

snacks. Vary the fruit and vegetables you eat every day, and aim for a rainbow of colours on your plate – the colours in fruit and vegetables are a result of the variety of antioxidant pigments they contain. Check the information on pages 56–57 so you know which are the best superfoods to include in your diet; for example, dark green leafy vegetables, apples, bananas, berries and carrots. You can even include dark chocolate (make sure it contains at least 70 percent cocoa solids) and three or four cups of coffee or cocoa a day.

Recipes Start adapting your own recipes to the principles of the gentle program. This means excluding added salt and using sugar sparingly. Most cookbook recipes are easy to adapt by replacing salt with herbs and black pepper for flavour. You can use honey in recipes instead of sugar if you need a sweetener.

Your long-term supplement regime

Continue taking your chosen selection of supplements from those I suggested on page 81. If your asthma is not fully controlled and you are not currently taking all the supplements in the desirable list, you may wish to add in those you have left out. Similarly, you may wish to add in one or more of the supplements in the optional list for additional benefits. Research supports their use at this level for gentle yet significant effects on asthma control. Full updates on latest research findings for these and other supplements is also available at www.naturalhealthguru.co.uk.

Your exercise routine

Having done the breath control exercises in the gentle program, you should have noticed an improvement in your lung function. Continue with these exercises and, as I recommended on page 96, try the Buteyko-based exercises I include in the moderate program. You can also try the yoga-based breathing exercises in the full-strength program – as long as you're benefiting from the gentle program diet you don't need to follow the low-sulfite or low-salicylate diets of the moderate and full-strength programs.

Aim to do at least 30 minutes of brisk exercise during most days, too; doing more as and when you feel ready. Increasing your level of physical exercise is important to maintain cardiorespiratory health, and to help you gain and maintain a healthy weight. Brisk walking, cycling, swimming, dancing, gardening, bowling and golf are all beneficial for lung health. And you don't have to complete your exercise all in one go – two daily sessions of 15 minutes or three daily sessions of 10 minutes are just as good for your long-term health as one longer session of 30 minutes. If exercise triggers your asthma, follow the advice I've given on pages 68–69 to help overcome this problem.

Your therapy program

The gentle program has shown you how to use aromatherapy to benefit your breathing, and introduced you to several other complementary techniques, including homeopathy, herbal medicine, meditation and the use of a negative ionizer. Continue to use the therapies that you have found most beneficial, and continue to consult an aromatherapist and homeopath, if you found their treatments helpful.

Monitoring your asthma

Continue to record your peak flow measurements on a chart such as that on page 77. This will tell you how you're doing, and give you early warning if your asthma control is starting to deteriorate. Ideally, you want to keep your peak flow readings within 20 percent of your personal best reading (see page 16). If your readings fall below 20 percent of your personal best, consult your doctor or asthma nurse.

breakfast recipes

full-of-goodness cereal

makes 1kg (2¼lb); 20 servings

400g/14oz/4 cups rolled oats
115g/4oz/1 scant cup sunflower seeds
115g/4oz/1¼ cups wheatgerm
115g/4oz/¾ cup Brazil nuts, chopped
115g/4oz/1 cup walnuts, chopped
100g/3½oz/½ cup brown sugar
150ml/5fl oz/²/₃ cup olive oil

1 Preheat the oven to
   150°C/300°F/Gas 2. Put the
   oats, seeds, wheatgerm, nuts
   and sugar in a bowl and mix.
2 Whisk the oil with 150ml/5fl oz/
   ²/₃ cup water. Stir into the dry
   ingredients and mix well.
3 Spread over several shallow
   roasting tins and bake for
   25–40 minutes, turning
   occasionally, until crisp and
   golden. Allow to cool. Store
   in an airtight container.

wholewheat, nuts and blueberries

serves 4

70g/2½oz/½ cup wholewheat
70g/2½oz/½ cup chopped mixed nuts
1 handful blueberries
Milk and honey, to serve

1 Put the wheat in a coffee
   grinder and grind to a
   medium texture.
2 Mix the wheat and nuts.
   Sprinkle the blueberries on top
   and serve with milk and honey.

sardine fishcakes

serves 4

4 sardine fillets, skinned and chopped
4 slices of bread, finely chopped
1 handful parsley, chopped
1 garlic clove, crushed
Juice of 1 lemon
1 egg, beaten
1 handful plain flour
4 tbsp olive oil
Freshly ground black pepper

1 Mix the sardines, bread,
   parsley, garlic and lemon juice
   in a bowl. Season with black
   pepper.
2 Add the egg and mix well.
   Make 12 small fishcakes from
   the sardine mixture and roll
   each one in flour.
3 Fry the fishcakes in the olive
   oil in a non-stick pan for 8–10
   minutes until golden. Drain on
   kitchen paper, then serve hot.

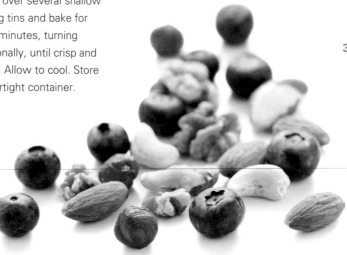

lunch recipes

minty mango and melon medley

serves 4

1 mango, peeled and cubed
1 Charentais melon, peeled and cubed
4 apricots, chopped
1 handful Brazil nuts
1 handful mint leaves, chopped
Juice and zest of 1 lime

1 Put all the ingredients except the lime juice and zest in a bowl. Mix well.
2 Drizzle with the lime juice and sprinkle with the zest. Divide between 4 glasses and serve.

mango oat-so smoothie

serves 4

2 mangos, peeled and chopped
450ml/16fl oz/1¾ cups low-fat bio yogurt
40g/1½oz/ ⅓ cup oats

1 Put the ingredients in a food processor and blend until smooth.
2 Divide between 4 glasses and serve.

anchovy and red pepper spread

serves 4

6 red peppers, deseeded and cut into quarters
50g/2oz tin anchovy fillets
1 onion, chopped
2 garlic cloves, crushed
2 tbsp olive oil
1 handful basil, chopped
1 handful parsley, chopped
8 slices wholegrain bread, toasted, to serve
Freshly ground black pepper

1 Preheat the oven to 200°C/400°F/Gas 6. Cook the peppers for 45 minutes. Allow to cool, discard the skins and chop the flesh.
2 Meanwhile, thoroughly rinse the anchovies, soak in water to remove excess salt, then drain.
3 Sauté the peppers, onion and garlic in the olive oil for 10 minutes. Add the anchovies and cook for a further 5 minutes. Season well with black pepper and leave to cool.
4 Blend the pepper mixture with the basil and parsley in a food processor until smooth. Serve on wholegrain bread.

gazpacho

serves 4

900g/2lb tomatoes, skinned, deseeded and chopped
½ cucumber, peeled and chopped
2 red peppers, deseeded and chopped
1 red chilli pepper, deseeded and chopped
3 garlic cloves, crushed
1 handful basil, chopped
2 tbsp balsamic vinegar
6 tbsp olive oil
300ml/10½fl oz/1¼ cups Low-Salicylate Vegetable Bouillon (see page 172)
Juice and zest of 1 unwaxed lemon
1 tsp honey
Freshly ground black pepper
Worcestershire sauce, to serve

1 Mix all the ingredients up to, and including, the olive oil and put in the refrigerator to marinate overnight.
2 Add the bouillon and lemon juice and zest and blend in a food processor until smooth.
3 Add the honey, season with black pepper and Worcestershire sauce, and serve chilled.

prawn and papaya citrus salad

serves 4

2 papayas, peeled, deseeded and
    chopped
1 pink grapefruit, peeled and chopped
1 orange (preferably a blood orange),
    peeled and chopped
450g/1lb king prawns, peeled and
    cooked
1 handful coriander leaves, chopped
Mixed salad leaves, to serve

For the dressing:
Juice and zest of 1 unwaxed lemon
1 tsp honey
1 tbsp soy sauce
2 tbsp walnut oil
Freshly ground black pepper

1 To make the dressing whisk
    together all the ingredients.
    Season well with black pepper.
2 Put the papaya, grapefruit,
    orange, prawns and coriander
    leaves in a bowl. Pour the
    dressing on top. Pile onto the
    mixed salad leaves and serve.

watercress, pear and pomegranate salad

serves 4

1 pomegranate, halved
4 pears, cored and chopped
1 handful walnut halves
1 bunch watercress

For the dressing:
1 garlic clove, crushed
2 tbsp balsamic vinegar
6 tbsp walnut oil
Freshly ground black pepper

1 To make the dressing whisk
    together all the ingredients.
    Season well with black pepper.
2 Hold the pomegranate over a
    bowl and bash with a wooden
    spoon to release the seeds.
    Add the pear, pomegranate and
    walnut. Pour the dressing on
    top. Pile the salad onto a bed of
    watercress and serve.

baked peppers with tomato stuffing

serves 4

4 red peppers, cut in half lengthways
    and deseeded
400g/14oz cherry tomatoes
2 tbsp olive oil
Freshly ground black pepper

For the dressing:
2 tbsp balsamic vinegar
4 tbsp extra virgin olive oil
1 handful basil, chopped
2 tsp soft brown sugar

1 Preheat the oven to
    180°C/350°F/Gas 4. Put the
    peppers on a non-stick baking
    sheet and fill with the cherry
    tomatoes. Drizzle with the
    olive oil and season with black
    pepper. Bake for 45 minutes.
2 Put the dressing ingredients in
    a screw-top jar and shake well.
3 Pour the dressing and the
    baking juices over the peppers
    and serve.

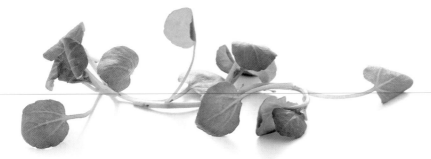

right: watercress, pear and pomegranate salad

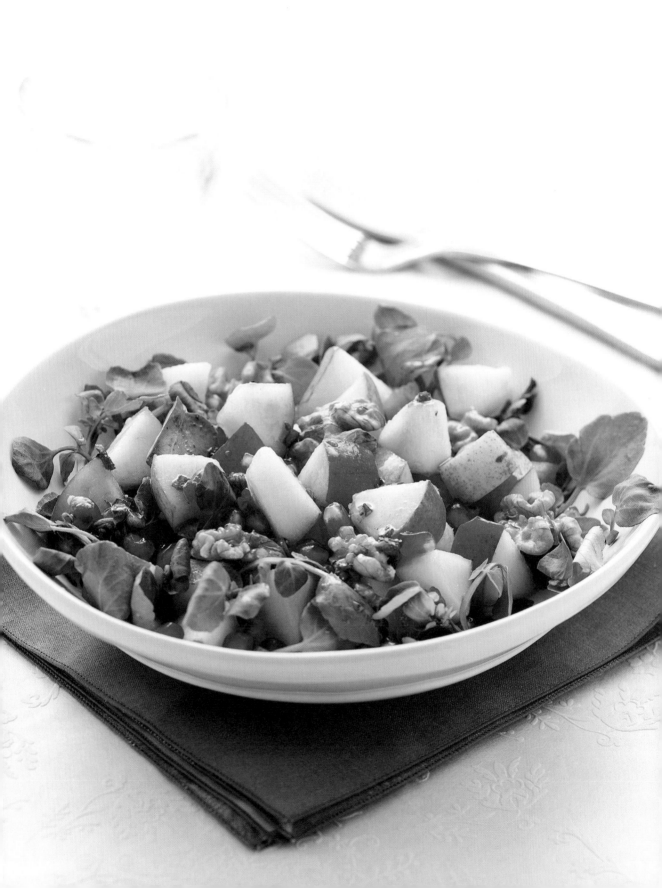

dinner recipes

aubergines parmesan

serves 4

1 large onion, sliced
4 garlic cloves, crushed
2 tbsp olive oil
700g/1lb 9oz tomatoes, skinned and
  chopped
2 tbsp tomato purée
125ml/4fl oz/½ cup dry white wine
1 handful mixed herbs, such as parsley,
  oregano and basil, chopped
2 large aubergines, sliced lengthways
225g/8oz mozzarella cheese, grated
Parmesan cheese, grated, to serve
Freshly ground black pepper

1   Preheat the oven to
    180°C/350°F/Gas 4. Sauté the
    onion and garlic in a little of the
    olive oil until starting to colour.
    Add the tomatoes, tomato
    purée, wine and herbs.

2   Simmer for 30 minutes, stirring
    occasionally. Season with
    black pepper.
3   Brush a pan with a little olive
    oil and lightly fry the aubergine
    slices in batches until soft and
    starting to colour. Re-brush
    the pan between batches,
    keeping the absorption of oil to
    a minimum.
4   Layer the tomato sauce,
    aubergine slices and mozzarella
    cheese in an ovenproof
    casserole dish, finishing with
    a layer of mozzarella. Sprinkle
    the Parmesan over the top
    and bake for 30 minutes,
    then serve.

creamy salmon in filo parcels

serves 4

125ml/4fl oz/½ cup low-fat crème fraîche
1 handful dill, chopped
8 sheets filo pastry
Olive oil, for brushing
4 salmon fillets, skinned
Freshly ground black pepper

1   Preheat the oven to
    200°C/400°F/Gas 6. Mix
    the crème fraîche and dill
    together and season well
    with black pepper.
2   Brush a sheet of pastry with
    olive oil. Place another sheet on
    top and brush with oil, too. Fold
    the layered pastry in half. Place
    one fillet of fish on one side of
    the pastry.
3   Cover the fish with a quarter
    of the dill sauce, then wrap the
    pastry round the fillet to make
    a neat parcel with the ends
    tucked under.
4   Place on a baking sheet and
    brush with olive oil. Repeat
    to make 4 parcels. Bake for
    20 minutes until golden brown.
    Serve immediately.

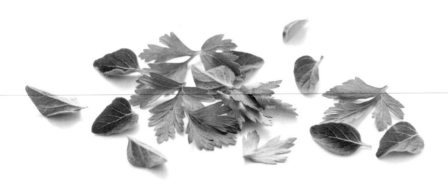

cod in green sauce

serves 4

4 garlic cloves, crushed
1 tbsp olive oil
4 cod steaks
Juice of 1 lemon
1 handful parsley, chopped
1 bay leaf
1 sprig rosemary
1 tbsp cornflour
125ml/4fl oz/½ cup fish stock (see page 112) or Low-Salicylate Vegetable Bouillon (see page 172) or water
120ml/4fl oz/½ cup dry white wine
4 potatoes, sliced
Freshly ground black pepper

1 Preheat the oven to 180°C/350°F/Gas 4. Sauté the garlic in the olive oil until starting to colour. Remove with a slotted spoon and reserve the oil.

2 Season the cod with black pepper and put in an ovenproof dish. Sprinkle with the lemon juice, fried garlic and herbs.

3 Blend the cornflour with the fish stock and wine and pour over the fish. Top with slices of potato and brush with the garlic oil. Bake for 30 minutes, then serve.

sole with red wine and grapes

serves 4

4 sole fillets, skinned
150ml/5fl oz/²/₃ cup light red wine, such as Beaujolais
1 bay leaf
1 spring onion, chopped
1 tbsp cornflour
150ml/5fl oz/²/₃ cup low-fat crème fraîche
100g/3½oz seedless black grapes
Freshly ground black pepper

1 Preheat the oven to 170°C/325°F/Gas 3. Put the rolled-up fillets in an ovenproof dish. Pour the wine and 4 tablespoons water over the top and add the bay leaf and spring onion. Season with black pepper.

2 Cover with foil and bake for 10 minutes. Remove the fish from the cooking liquid and keep warm. Strain the liquid into a pan.

3 Mix the cornflour with a little water and stir into the liquid. Simmer over a gentle heat, stirring gently until the mixture thickens.

4 Remove from the heat and stir in the crème fraîche and grapes. Warm through, pour over the top of the fish and serve.

baked orange and rosemary trout

serves 4

4 whole trout, cleaned
2 oranges, peeled and sliced
4 sprigs rosemary
1 tsp coriander seeds, crushed
Freshly ground black pepper

1 Preheat the oven to 190°C/375°F/Gas 5. Stuff the trout with the orange slices, rosemary and coriander seeds. Season well with black pepper.

2 Wrap in foil and bake for 20 minutes, then serve.

mackerel with mustard and herbs

. . . .

serves 4

4 whole mackerel, cleaned
4 tsp wholegrain mustard
1 handful mixed herbs, such as lemon
 thyme, parsley, chives or basil,
 chopped
Juice and zest of 1 unwaxed lemon
100ml/3½fl oz/scant ½ cup white wine

1 Make 4–5 slashes on each side
 of the mackerel.
2 Mix the mustard with the
 herbs, lemon juice and zest.
 Rub into the mackerel and put
 any remaining mixture inside
 the fish.
3 Put the fish in a shallow dish
 and pour the white wine over
 the top. Leave to marinate in
 the fridge for at least
 1 hour, turning occasionally.
4 Grill for 5–8 minutes on each
 side, then serve.

lamb alla romana

. . . .

serves 4

4 lamb steaks
2 sprigs rosemary
4 tbsp olive oil
4 anchovy fillets
1 handful basil, chopped
4 garlic cloves, crushed
1 tbsp red wine vinegar
Freshly ground black pepper

1 Season the lamb well with
 black pepper. Strip the leaves
 from the rosemary sprigs and
 pound together with the oil,
 anchovies, basil and garlic. Mix
 with the red wine vinegar.
2 Sauté the lamb over a high heat
 to seal in the juices. Pour the
 anchovy and vinegar mixture
 over the meat and cook for
 5–10 minutes. Serve
 immediately.

coq au vin rouge

. . . .

serves 4

4 chicken breasts, skinned and boned
1 garlic clove, crushed
8 shallots, peeled
8 button mushrooms, sliced
1 tbsp olive oil
1 tbsp brandy
375ml/13fl oz/1½ cups red Burgundy
 wine
1 bouquet garni (1 bay leaf, 1 sprig each
 thyme and rosemary, tied together)
1 handful parsley, chopped
Freshly ground black pepper

1 Sauté the chicken, garlic,
 shallots and mushrooms in a
 little of the olive oil until starting
 to colour.
2 Pour the brandy over the
 chicken and set alight. As the
 flames die, add the wine and
 bouquet garni. Cover and cook
 gently for 30 minutes.
3 Remove the bouquet garni,
 season with black pepper,
 sprinkle with parsley and serve.

herby orange chicken

. . . .

serves 4

1 large onion, chopped
2 garlic cloves, crushed
2 tbsp olive oil
1 chicken, skinned
300ml/10½fl oz/1¼ cups chicken stock
 or Low-Salicylate Vegetable Bouillon
 (see page 172)
125ml/4fl oz/½ cup white wine
1 handful parsley, chopped
1 handful chives, chopped
1 handful coriander, chopped
1 handful mint, chopped
Juice and zest of 2 large unwaxed
 oranges
1 handful walnut halves
Freshly ground black pepper

1 Sweat the onion and garlic in
 the olive oil in a flame-proof
 dish until soft. Add the chicken,
 stock and white wine and
 season with black pepper.
2 Bring to the boil, cover and
 simmer for 1 hour, basting the
 chicken regularly.
3 Add the herbs, orange juice and
 zest and walnuts and simmer
 for a further 30 minutes. Serve
 immediately.

right: herby orange chicken

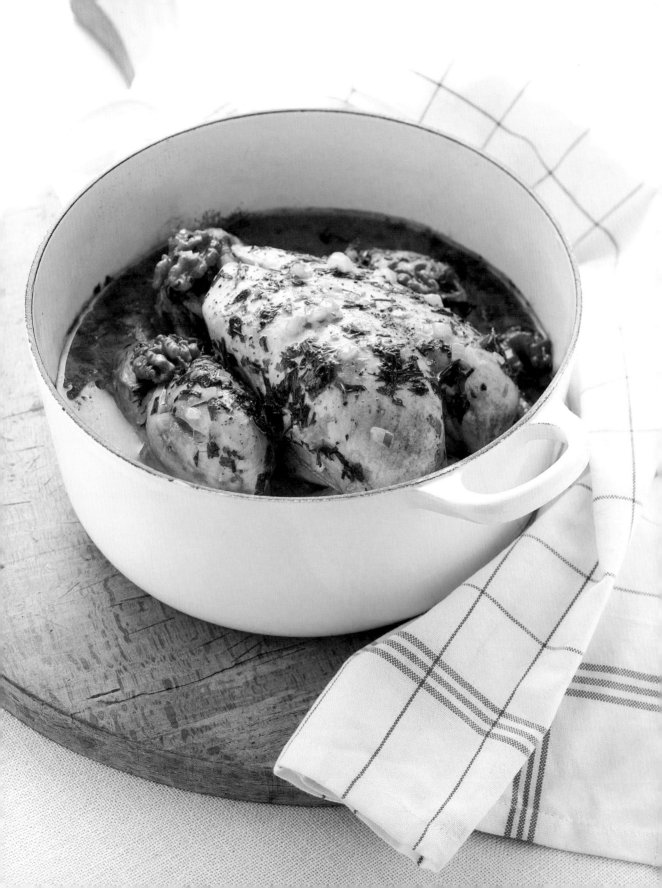

dessert recipes

pears in citrus red wine

. . . .

serves 4

375ml/13fl oz/1½ cups red wine
85g/3oz/⅓ cup sugar
Juice and zest of 1 unwaxed orange
Juice and zest of 1 unwaxed lemon
10cm/4in length of cinnamon stick
4 ripe but firm pears, peeled, cored and
 halved

1 Put the red wine, sugar, orange
 and lemon juice and zest in a
 pan with the cinnamon stick.
 Heat gently to dissolve the
 sugar. Simmer for 1 minute.
2 Put the pear halves in the
 wine. Cover and cook for 5–10
 minutes. Turn frequently during
 cooking. Use a slotted spoon to
 transfer the pears to a bowl.
3 Boil the wine until it has
 reduced by half. Pour it over
 the top of the pears and chill
 before serving.

fruit crumble

. . . .

serves 4

700g/1lb 9oz mixed fruit, such as
 apples, plums and rhubarb, chopped
Sprinkling of caster sugar (optional)
100g/3½oz/⅔ cup wholewheat flour
55g/2oz butter
55g/2oz/ ⅓ cup brown sugar

1 Preheat the oven to
 190°C/375°F/Gas 5. Put the
 fruit in an ovenproof dish and
 sprinkle with the sugar, if using.
2 Rub together the flour and
 butter to make the crumble
 topping. Stir in the brown
 sugar, then sprinkle the
 crumble mixture over the
 fruit. Bake for 30 minutes,
 then serve.

bittersweet fruit compote

. . . .

serves 4

200g/7oz/scant 1 cup sugar
225g/8oz kumquats, sliced
225g/8oz clementines, peeled and
 segmented
115g/4oz black seedless grapes
115g/4oz green seedless grapes
115g/4oz cranberries

1 Put the sugar and 250ml/
 9fl oz/1 cup water in a pan and
 simmer over a low heat. Add
 the kumquat slices, cover and
 poach gently for 15 minutes.
2 Add the clementine segments
 and grapes and cook for a
 further 5 minutes, turning
 regularly. Add the cranberries
 and cook for a further
 5 minutes.
3 Use a slotted spoon to transfer
 the fruit to a bowl. Serve hot or
 cold, with the syrup poured on
 top, if you wish.

right: oranges in caramel

oranges in caramel

serves 4

150g/5½oz/⅔ cup sugar
400ml/14fl oz/1⅔ cups boiling water
4 large oranges
2 tbsp Grand Marnier or Cointreau
   orange liqueur (optional)

1 Place the sugar in a saucepan
with 50ml/2fl oz/¼ cup water
and heat gently until the sugar
dissolves. Brush down the
sides of the pan with hot water
to prevent crystals forming.

2 Bring to the boil and simmer
until the syrup turns golden
caramel. Immediately plunge
the base of the saucepan in
boiling water to prevent
further darkening.

3 Add 350ml/12fl oz/scant 1½
cups boiling water to the pan
and heat gently until all the
caramel dissolves.

4 Meanwhile, remove the zest
from 2 of the oranges and
add to the caramel. Then peel
and discard the pith from all
the oranges.

5 Put the oranges in the caramel,
cover and poach them gently
for 20–25 minutes, turning
them occasionally. Add the
orange liqueur, if using, and
chill before serving.

tangy apple swirl

serves 4

4 cooking apples, peeled and chopped
Juice and zest of 1 unwaxed lemon
25g/1oz butter
50g/1¾oz/¼ cup brown sugar
290ml/10fl oz/heaped 1 cup low-fat bio
   yogurt
4 mint sprigs

1 Put all the ingredients except
the yogurt and mint in a pan
and cook gently, stirring
occasionally, until the apples
are soft. Mash with a fork and
leave to cool.

2 Spoon alternate layers of the
yogurt and apple purée into
4 tall glasses. With a knife,
swirl the mixtures together and
serve with a mint sprig on top.

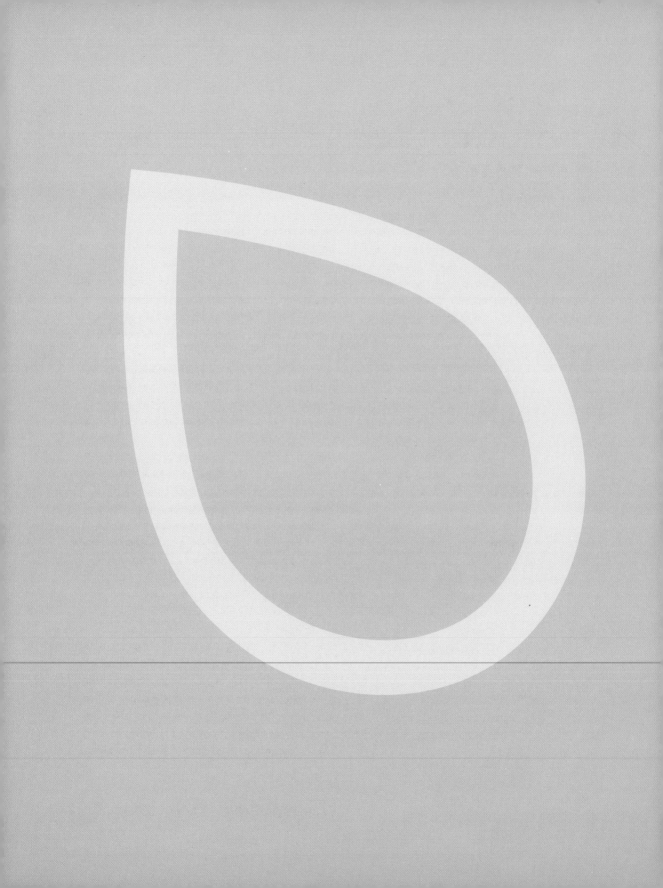

introducing the moderate program

The moderate program is a more advanced dietary and lifestyle plan for people with asthma. It's designed to eliminate dietary sulfites (see pages 46–47), which may be triggering your asthma. If, by the end of the program, your asthma has improved, it's likely that you have a sulfite sensitivity – avoiding sulfites in the future should play a key part in your asthma management. If your asthma hasn't improved, this suggests that sulfites are not the culprit.

I'd advise you to follow the moderate program if, having followed the gentle program, you still have troublesome asthma symptoms; or if you know or strongly suspect you have a sensitivity to sulfites (the questionnaire on pages 75–76 can help you decide). However, if the gentle program worked for you and you're happy to continue following its principles, then please do so.

The moderate program diet

The daily food plans eliminate foods that have a high content of sulfites, whether naturally present or added as a food preservative. To remind yourself about sulfites, please re-read pages 46–47. You will need to avoid all processed, canned, frozen and dried commercial products. If it's essential to use a convenience food product, check the labels and avoid those that contain the additives described on page 46. I recommend that you buy organic products – these are least likely to have sulfites added (although some products, such as organic grapes and wine, will contain natural sulfites).

Making your own juices Because most shop-bought juices contain sulfites, I strongly recommend that you invest in a juicer to prepare your own delicious fruit and vegetable juices at home. Freshly prepared juice has a creamy texture and is richer in antioxidants, vitamins and minerals than those that are commercially processed. Juicing also concentrates the beneficial, anti-asthma nutrients found in fruit and vegetables. For example, you'd have to eat 450g (1lb) of raw carrots to obtain as many carotenoids as you get in 100ml (3½fl oz) of carrot juice. The power of concentration is especially important in the case of apple juice – a glass a day provides a potent quercetin-rich drink. Research shows that children who drink apple juice at least once a day are almost half as likely to have asthma as those drinking apple juice less than once a month.

You can combine juices, such as tomato and celery, or apple and mango, to make interesting, delicious drinks. You can also make an antioxidant-rich lemonade by mixing a juiced lemon (plus peel) with sparkling mineral water and a little honey.

There are a few important rules to follow when juicing at home. Use only organic fruit and vegetables for juicing – others may have been subjected to a sulfite wash to prolong their shelf-life. Where possible, buy locally grown, harvest-fresh produce for maximum antioxidant content – join a local organic box scheme or a co-operative that supports small producers in your area. Check out local farmer's markets, too. Another option is to use freshly frozen organic produce, such as strawberries, raspberries, blueberries and cranberries

Shopping list

This list shows you the foods you should base your shopping lists on. Always buy fresh organic products.

drinks
ground coffee, mineral water, camomile tea, green/black/white tea

dairy products
butter (unsalted), low-fat cottage cheese, fromage frais, low-fat bio yogurt, mascarpone, mozzarella, low-fat crème fraîche, skimmed/semi-skimmed milk, single and double cream, sour cream, sour milk, ricotta

fruit
apples (dessert and cooking), apricots (fresh, and dried without sulfites), bananas, blackberries, blackcurrants, blueberries, cranberries, dates (dried without sulfites), figs (dried without sulfites), grapefruit*, kiwi fruit, lemons, limes, mango, oranges, papaya, pears, pineapple, plums, pomegranate, raspberries, redcurrants, strawberries
*Check for interactions between grapefruit and your medication

vegetables and salad stuff
avocado, aubergine, beetroot, broccoli, cabbage (dark green and white), carrots, celery, chard, courgettes, corn-on-the-cob, cucumber, garden peas, lettuce, kale, mixed salad leaves, mushrooms, onions, potatoes (new), red peppers, spinach, spring onions, sweetcorn, sweet potatoes, tomatoes (including cherry), watercress

nuts and seeds
almonds, Brazils, walnuts; sunflower, pumpkin, sesame

herbs and spices
allspice, black pepper, chillies (green and red), coriander leaf, coriander seed, cumin, dill, garlic, mint, mixed spice, parsley, rosemary, sage, tarragon, thyme

oils and condiments
extra virgin olive oil (for drizzling and dressings), home-made chutneys made with allowed ingredients, olive oil (for cooking), rapeseed oil, salt, walnut oil

grains
(always choose unbleached, wholegrain organic products) barley flakes, bran flakes, breakfast cereals without dried fruit or coconut, bulgur wheat, couscous, plain pasta (fresh or dried; for example, tagliatelle) porridge oats, rice (brown, red, risotto, white, wild), rye flakes, wheat flakes

proteins
(always choose fresh unprocessed meat and fish) beef tenderloin, chicken, crab, duck, halibut, lamb, lobster, mackerel, omega-3-enriched eggs, prawns, salmon (smoked and fillet), shellfish that haven't had a sulfite wash, tuna, turkey

miscellaneous
bread soda, caster sugar, low-sulfite jam and marmalade without added pectin or gelatin (see page 133), honey, white and brown sugar

(freezing preserves their nutrients). Some fruits such as bananas and avocados are difficult to juice as they are so dense – instead you can mash or blend them and stir them into other fruit juices to make thick smoothies. You can also dilute juices with mineral water for a thirst-quenching drink.

Making your own stock and soup Whenever you have bones left over from a dish that includes turkey, duck, chicken, lamb, fish or even lobster, boil them up with onions and herbs to make a delicious broth. Freeze picked-over chicken carcases until you have four to six that you can boil up in a large saucepan to make a super-concentrated, well-flavoured stock.

Stock can be used as the basis for wonderfully nutritious stews, sauces, gravies and soups. To make home-made soup, all you need to do is sauté some vegetables, then cover them with stock, add some fresh herbs and garlic, and simmer until the vegetables are tender. You can also use juices to make tasty soups, such as carrot and orange – simply sauté some onion and carrots, and then simmer them in carrot and orange juice with fresh herbs, such as sage or coriander. If you want a smooth consistency, blend the soup in a food processor before serving. I include home-made soup ideas in several of the lunches in the moderate program, but you don't have to follow my suggestions – just use the vegetables you have.

The moderate program exercise routine

The breathing exercises I suggest for the moderate program are based on the Buteyko method (see pages 38–39). These are designed to encourage breathing through your nose rather than your mouth to direct air toward the lower parts of your lungs. They also encourage shallow breathing, which reduces the amount of air you take in if you habitually hyperventilate (overbreathe). This helps a significant number of people

The moderate program supplements

The supplements I recommend on the moderate program are similar to those in the gentle program but, where appropriate, at a higher, more therapeutic dose. Those in the recommended list are most likely to have a beneficial effect on your asthma symptoms. Those in the optional list have the potential to improve your symptoms further. You can find information about these supplements and their benefits on pages 60–61.

recommended daily supplements

- Vitamin C (1000mg)
- Vitamin E (400mg)
- Vitamin B12 (100mcg, preferably via a sub-lingual tablet)
- Lycopene carotenoid complex (15mg)
- Magnesium (400mg)
- Selenium (100mcg)
- Omega-3 fish oils (2x1g fish oil capsules, each supplying 180mg EPA + 120mg DHA; DHA-only blends are recommended during pregnancy)
- Pycnogenol (100mg)

optional daily supplements (these provide additional health benefits)

- Co-enzyme Q10 (60mg)
- Quercetin (500mg, three times a day before food)
- Bromelain (100mg, twice daily to enhance quercetin absorption)
- N-acetyl-l-cysteine (NAC) (100mg, three times a day)
- Reishi (1000mg or 500mg, twice a day)
- Digestive enzymes (mixed; 2 capsules before meals)
- Probiotics (in the form of fermented milk drinks, bio yogurt or supplements)

with asthma to control their symptoms and reduce their dependence on a reliever inhaler.

Take aerobic exercise As well as the breathing exercises, you should do at least 15 minutes of brisk aerobic exercise every day. Rather than exercising until you feel slightly breathless (as in the gentle program), I want you to exert yourself less – don't exercise to the point where you have to open your mouth to breathe. Instead continue to breathe through your nose according to the Buteyko principles. If you have problems with exercise-induced asthma, read the tips on pages 68–69 and use your reliever inhaler 15 minutes before starting your daily exercise routine.

To help maintain a good level of physical exercise, I recommend that you buy a small pedometer to clip to your clothes while following the moderate program.

This measures the number of steps you take each day and acts as a great motivator to improve your general level of activity. The ideal aim is to take 10,000 steps a day. If you are unfit, or have exercise-induced asthma, aim for 5,000 steps initially and slowly work up. Keep a record of the number of paces you take each day so you have a tangible record of your progress.

The moderate program therapies

The complementary therapy regime for the moderate program is based on reflexology. During the second week of the program, I show you some other approaches from a variety of therapies – you can try them all and find which techniques suit you best. Please look at days seven and fourteen of the program now so that you can book appointments with the appropriate therapists.

the moderate program day one

Daily menu

- **Breakfast: toast made with Low-Sulfite Soda Bread (see page 132). Low-Sulfite Raspberry Jam (see page 133)**

- **Morning snack: a large apple**

- **Lunch: bowl of mixed salad leaves drizzled with olive oil and fresh lemon juice, and sprinkled with seeds. Cottage cheese mixed with fresh pineapple. Bread roll**

- **Afternoon snack: handful of Brazil nuts**

- **Dinner: Ratatouille (stir-fry onions, garlic, courgettes and aubergine, then add tomatoes, herbs and home-made stock (see page 112). Brown rice. Almond-stuffed Plums (see page 40)**

- **Drinks: 570ml/20fl oz/scant 2¹/₃ cups semi-skimmed or skimmed milk. Three or four cups of ground coffee. Unlimited green/black/white tea, camomile tea and mineral water. Freshly squeezed apple juice (and other freshly squeezed juices)**

- **Supplements: see page 113**

Daily breathing exercise

Today you're going to learn how to measure your resting pulse rate – you need to know how to do this for some of the later exercises in the moderate program. As long as you haven't recently used a reliever inhaler and you aren't taking any medication that affects your heart rate, a resting pulse rate of 60–69 shows good cardiorespiratory fitness (or that you're experienced in the Buteyko method). A resting pulse rate of 70–79 is considered fair; and a resting pulse rate of 80 or more suggests you are overbreathing (hyperventilating) or that your cardiorespiratory fitness is poor. Usually, only trained athletes or Buteyko adepts have a resting pulse rate that is naturally (and safely) below 60 beats per minute. If your resting pulse rate is unexpectedly below 60, or above 90, I advise you to consult your doctor before continuing this program.

Measuring your carotid pulse

1 Relax, breathing normally, for at least five minutes.
2 Rest your fingertips (not your thumb) on the side of your neck underneath your jaw. Count the beats over 15 seconds and then multiply by four.
3 Make a note of your pulse rate.

Reflexology

Reflexology can reduce stress and upper-body tension and relieve asthma. Today's technique stimulates the lung reflexes at the base of your three middle fingers.

Palm press

1 Press your upper parts of your palms firmly together.
2 Hold for 10 seconds, relax and repeat. Do this often or whenever you feel asthma symptoms coming on. If you've got nasal congestion, spread your fingers wide apart to balance your sinuses while performing this technique.

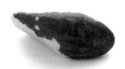
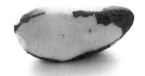

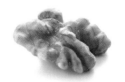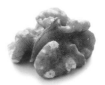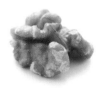

day two

Daily menu

- **Breakfast: Low-Sulfite Muesli (see page 132) with chopped fruit**

- **Morning snack: a large apple**

- **Lunch: Avocado Dip (see page 134). Carrot, celery, cucumber and pepper cut into sticks or strips. Toast made with Low-Sulfite Soda Bread (see page 132)**

- **Afternoon snack: handful of walnuts**

- **Dinner: roast crown of turkey with Cranberry Sauce (see box). Roast potatoes. Broccoli. Carrots. A handful of cherries or berries**

- **Drinks: 570ml/20fl oz/scant 2¹/₃ cups semi-skimmed or skimmed milk. Three or four cups of ground coffee. Unlimited green/black/white tea, camomile tea and mineral water. Freshly squeezed apple juice (and other freshly squeezed juices)**

- **Supplements: see page 113**

You'll notice that each daily menu in the moderate program contains a large apple and some freshly squeezed apple juice (make this at home) – the flavonoid antioxidants in apples can reduce your asthma symptoms.

Daily breathing exercise

The Buteyko method promotes breathing through your nose at all times – today's exercise helps you to get into this habit.

Nostril breathing

1 Sit comfortably in an upright posture – imagine a string attached to the top of your head pulling you up straight as your upper body relaxes. Don't tense your shoulders.

2 Breathe in slowly and gently through your nose, then out again. Find your own rhythm.

3 From now on, regularly check that you're breathing in and out through your nostrils all the time in everyday life.

Reflexology

People with allergic asthma can benefit from massage of the adrenal gland reflex on the palms.

The best way to apply pressure to this area is with a golf ball.

Palm massage

1 Clasp a golf ball between your two hands, with your fingers interlinked.

2 Roll the golf ball over the fleshy part of your palms beneath the inner edge of each thumb. This targets both your adrenal reflexes in one go.

3 Perform the golf-ball massage for 30 seconds, then rest for 30 seconds and repeat for five minutes overall. Do this twice, and preferably four times today.

Cranberry sauce
You should avoid shop-bought cranberry sauce because it contains sulfites, but you can easily make your own: chop 225g/8oz cranberries in a food processor and then boil in water for five minutes with the zest and juice of an unwaxed orange and 40g/1½oz caster sugar. You can also add a sprinkling of mixed spice.

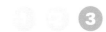

the moderate program day three

Daily menu

- **Breakfast: Scrambled Eggs with Red Pepper and Tomato (see page 133). Toast made with Low-Sulfite Soda Bread (see page 132)**

- **Morning snack: a large apple**

- **Lunch: home-made turkey and vegetable soup (see page 112). Bread roll**

- **Afternoon snack: handful of Brazil nuts**

- **Dinner: Potato and Smoked Salmon Pancakes (see page 138). Spinach. Sweetcorn. Slices of red grapefruit and orange**

- **Drinks: 570ml/20fl oz/scant 2¹⁄₃ cups semi-skimmed or skimmed milk. Three or four cups of ground coffee. Unlimited green/black/white tea, camomile tea and mineral water. Freshly squeezed apple juice (and other freshly squeezed juices)**

- **Supplements: see page 113**

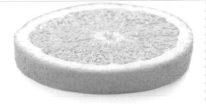

Today's menu includes omega-3 enriched eggs, and omega-3 rich salmon. By increasing your intake of omega-3s and reducing your intake of omega-6 essential fatty acids, you're reducing the production of inflammatory chemicals in your body. This can significantly improve your asthma symptoms. However, a few people are intolerant to fish or eggs. If you find your asthma symptoms are related to eating these foods, exchange them for other omega-3 rich foods instead: walnuts, pumpkin seeds, soy beans, flax seed (linseed) oil and rapeseed oil. Vegetarian omega-3 oil supplements made from algae sources are also available.

Daily breathing exercise

The Buteyko method uses the following technique, called tipping, to help clear blocked nasal passages.

Tipping

1 Breathe in gently through your nose. Breathe out and gently hold your nose between your finger and thumb. Keep your mouth closed.

2 Hold your breath and tip your head backward and forward six times.

3 Release your nose and, still keeping your mouth closed, breathe in slowly through both nostrils.

4 Use this technique whenever your nose feels blocked. You can also try pinching your nostrils together for a few seconds to help clear your nasal passages.

Reflexology

The lung reflexes in your feet are situated on the ball of each foot (see the foot maps on page 34). Today, I'd like you to practise balancing on the balls of your feet to stimulate your lung reflexes. You may also find this technique helpful when you feel your asthma symptoms starting.

Stimulating the lung reflexes

1 Balance on the balls of your feet for 10 seconds, then relax back down onto your heels and repeat.

2 Do this for five minutes and repeat three more times throughout the day.

day four

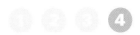

Daily menu

- **Breakfast: smoothie made by whizzing a banana, some blueberries, some low-fat bio yogurt and a handful of porridge oats in a food processor**

- **Morning snack: a large apple**

- **Lunch: cold turkey. Bowl of mixed salad leaves drizzled with olive oil and fresh lemon juice, and sprinkled with seeds. Freshly boiled beetroot (no vinegar). Sulfite-Free Coleslaw (see page 135). Bread roll**

- **Afternoon snack: handful of walnuts**

- **Dinner: Duck à l'Orange (see page 137). Red Rice Pilaf (see page 137). Courgettes. Dark green cabbage. Minted Apples and Berries (see page 141)**

- **Drinks: 570ml/20fl oz/scant 2¹/₃ cups semi-skimmed or skimmed milk. Three or four cups of ground coffee. Unlimited green/black/white tea, camomile tea and mineral water. Freshly squeezed apple juice (and other freshly squeezed juices)**

- **Supplements: see page 113**

Daily breathing exercise

People with asthma tend to overbreathe and have lower than normal levels of carbon dioxide in their blood (see page 39). When you breathe more than normal, you are unable to hold your breath for as long as you should. Today's exercise, called the control pause (CP), monitors your level of hyperventilation. This is the length of time you can comfortably hold your breath after breathing out normally. Don't be tempted to hold your breath for longer than is comfortable, or you'll be forced to gasp for air, which goes against the aims of breath control. Many people have a CP of below 20 when they first start the Buteyko technique, but it improves as you become more proficient. A CP of 30 is acceptable, but your goal is a CP of at least 40, and preferably 60 or more, which is classed as excellent.

Measuring your control pause

1 To measure your CP take two gentle breaths, then breathe out normally (don't try to completely empty your lungs).

2 Using a stopwatch time how many seconds you can hold your breath until you feel uncomfortable. The number of seconds is your CP reading.

3 At this point start breathing again through your nose. You should be able to resume normal breathing without effort and without gasping for air.

Reflexology

Today, I show you how to stimulate the lung and bronchial tube reflexes on the fronts of your ears. This technique can help when you feel your asthma symptoms starting to come on.

Ear massage

1 Gently place your right index finger inside your right ear canal with your nail facing forward.

2 Bring the pad of your finger back out and slightly downward. Firmly massage the part of your ear that lies between your ear canal and the rim of your ear. Do this for one minute.

3 Repeat with your left index finger and your left ear. Do this often today, whenever you remember.

the moderate program day five

Daily menu

- **Breakfast: toast made with Low-Sulfite Soda Bread (see page 132). Low-Sulfite Old-English Marmalade (see page 133)**

- **Morning snack: a large apple**

- **Lunch: slices of mozzarella cheese sprinkled with pomegranate seeds. Sulfite-Free Coleslaw (see page 135). Bowl of mixed salad leaves drizzled with olive oil and fresh lemon juice, and sprinkled with seeds**

- **Afternoon snack: handful of Brazil nuts**

- **Dinner: Couscous with Roast Vegetables and Tomato Sauce (see page 139). Spinach. Platter of tropical fruit, such as kiwi fruit, papaya, mango and pineapple**

- **Drinks: 570ml/20fl oz/scant 2¹/₃ cups semi-skimmed or skimmed milk. Three or four cups of ground coffee. Unlimited green/black/white tea, camomile tea and mineral water. Freshly squeezed apple juice (and other freshly squeezed juices)**

- **Supplements: see page 113**

Daily breathing exercise

The Buteyko method promotes shallow rather than deep breathing. Shallow breathing is the most important, yet most difficult type of breathing to master, and should produce a feeling of slight air hunger. Practise the exercises on the following pages on an empty stomach, or at least two hours after eating. Wear loose, comfortable clothing. If any breathing techniques make you feel dizzy, sick or anxious, or bring on palpitations, stop immediately and consult a Buteyko practitioner before continuing the program.

Shallow breathing

1 Breathe in and out through your nose for five minutes – make your breaths as gentle and shallow as you possibly can. Keep your mouth closed all the time.

2 Place your index finger beneath your nostrils – if you can feel your breath on your finger, you're breathing too deeply.

Reflexology

Today, I show you how to stimulate the lung and bronchial

Sea spray

Spending time by the sea is beneficial for people with asthma. Sea spray is rich in minerals and negative ions, while off-shore breezes are pollen-free. To capture some of these benefits, cleanse and humidify your nose daily with a purified seawater spray – these are widely available in pharmacies.

tube reflexes that lie behind your ears. This technique can help generally but you can also use it any time you feel your asthma symptoms starting.

Ear massage 2

1 Place your right index finger behind your right ear in the vertical crease where your ear joins your scalp.

2 Massage the back of your ear at the midpoint of this crease for one minute.

3 Repeat with your left finger behind your left ear. Do this often today, whenever you remember.

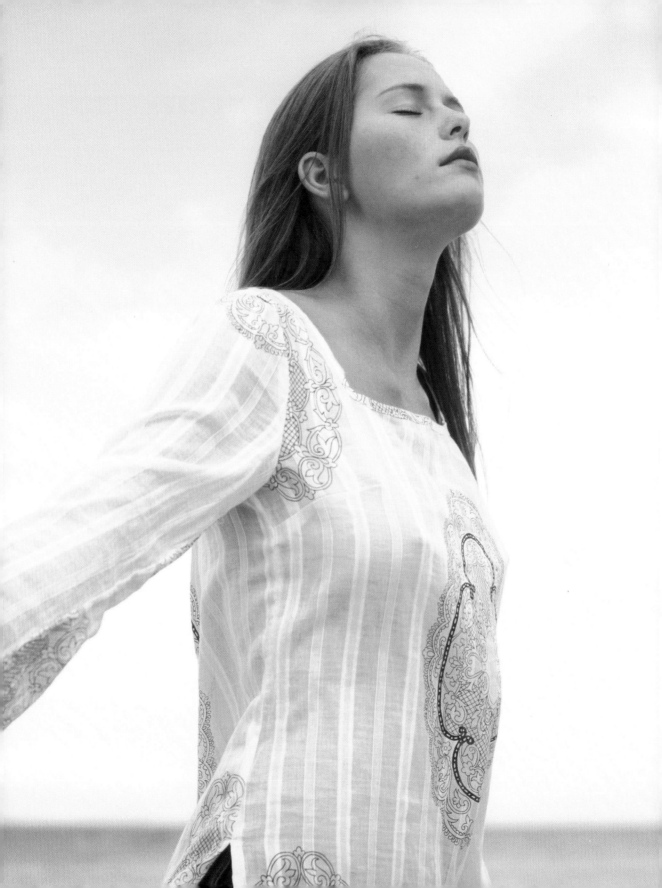

the moderate program day six

Daily menu

- **Breakfast: Low-Sulfite Muesli (see page 132) with chopped fruit**
- **Morning snack: a large apple**
- **Lunch: home-made vegetable soup, such as carrot and orange (see page 112). Bowl of mixed salad leaves drizzled with olive oil and fresh lemon juice, and sprinkled with seeds. Bread roll**
- **Afternoon snack: handful of walnuts**
- **Dinner: Spicy Mackerel (see page 137). Boiled new potatoes. Carrots. Dark green leaves, such as chard or kale. Apple Fool (mix together low-fat bio yogurt and freshly cooked apple purée)**
- **Drinks: 570ml/20fl oz/scant 2¹/₃ cups semi-skimmed or skimmed milk. Three or four cups of ground coffee. Unlimited green/black/white tea, camomile tea and mineral water. Freshly squeezed apple juice (and other freshly squeezed juices)**
- **Supplements: see page 113**

If you don't want to make your own muesli, select an organic ready-made one that doesn't contain dried fruit, coconut or other sulfite sources. You can liven up muesli with chopped fresh fruit such as banana or antioxidant-rich berries. Add fromage frais or bio yogurt for extra calcium.

Daily breathing exercise

Repeat the five-minute shallow breathing technique you learned yesterday, followed by the control pause test from day four. Do this four times in a row. This should take around 25 minutes and you should find that your CP improves. Repeat this intensive session two or three times a day, every day. Your CP should improve by one or two seconds per week. Your asthma should improve, too.

Reflexology

Today, I'd like you to spend 10 minutes performing the reflexology routine described on page 33. From now on do this once or twice a day. Also stimulate the reflexes on your hands, feet and ears as described earlier this week.

Health benefits of pineapple

Bromelain, an enzyme found in the stem of pineapple plants, has an anti-inflammatory action that helps to reduce pain, swelling and inflammation. Its enzyme action also helps to break down mucus so that it's easier to shift. Bromelain is especially helpful for reducing allergic symptoms in the nasal passages and sinuses. In one study, 83 percent of people taking it for sinusitis enjoyed resolution of nasal swelling and inflammation compared with half of those taking a placebo.

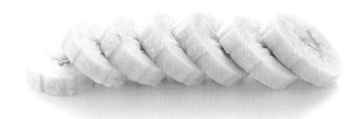

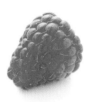

day seven

Daily menu

- **Breakfast: toast made with Low-Sulfite Soda Bread (see page 132). Low-Sulfite Raspberry Jam (see page 133)**

- **Morning snack: a large apple**

- **Lunch: Crab and Orange Salad (see page 134). Bowl of mixed salad leaves drizzled with olive oil and fresh lemon juice, and sprinkled with seeds. Bread roll**

- **Afternoon snack: handful of Brazil nuts**

- **Dinner: Beef Tenderloin with Brown Mushrooms and Potatoes (see page 137). Stir-fried mixed vegetables. Apricot and Walnut Crumble (see page 141)**

- **Drinks: 570ml/20fl oz/scant 2¹/₃ cups semi-skimmed or skimmed milk. Three or four cups of ground coffee. Unlimited green/black/white tea, camomile tea and mineral water. Freshly squeezed apple juice (and other freshly squeezed juices)**

- **Supplements: see page 113**

Daily breathing exercise

Today I'd like you to check that you are doing the reduced breathing exercise correctly: your pulse should go down (or stay the same) and your control pause (CP; see day four) should go up.

Monitoring your pulse and CP

1 Measure and write down your pulse rate and your CP (see days one and four).

2 Practise the reduced, shallow breathing exercises that you learned on day five for 10 minutes.

3 Breathe normally and gently through your nose for five minutes, then measure your pulse rate and your CP again.

4 Compare your pulse rate and CP readings from before and after the breathing exercise. If your pulse rate has gone down and your CP has gone up, you are practising the technique correctly. If your pulse rate has gone up and your CP has gone down, you may need help in perfecting the technique – I advise you to seek advice from a Buteyko practitioner.

Consulting a reflexologist

Having followed the moderate program for one week, you should have started to notice an improvement in your asthma symptoms. You've learned some basic reflexology techniques that are beneficial for people with asthma, and now I'd like you to visit a professional reflexologist. He or she will be able to show you further techniques to use at home. Most reflexologists work on reflexes in the feet, but some may use reflexes on your hands or ears, too. For the feet, after removing your footwear, you'll be asked to relax on a seat or couch with your feet raised. The therapist will dust your feet with powder and then massage your reflexes using their fingers and thumbs. Reflexologists focus on areas of tenderness and grittiness to diagnose distant problems in the body before using therapeutic massage to open up blocked nerve pathways and promote the flow of energy. A session usually lasts from 45 to 60 minutes. Book yourself in for four weekly sessions. To find a reflexologist, check the resources on pages 175.

the moderate program day eight

Daily menu

- **Breakfast: porridge made with rolled oats and topped with banana and flaked almonds**

- **Morning snack: a large apple**

- **Lunch: cold beef. Bowl of mixed salad leaves drizzled with olive oil and fresh lemon juice and sprinkled with seeds. Freshly boiled beetroot (no vinegar). Sulfite-Free Coleslaw (see page 134). Bread roll**

- **Afternoon snack: handful of walnuts**

- **Dinner: Tagliatelle with Herby Lemon and Walnut Butter (see page 138). Mixed salad leaves drizzled with olive oil. Frozen berries, such as raspberries and blueberries, puréed and mixed with fromage frais**

- **Drinks: 570ml/20fl oz/scant 2¹/₃ cups semi-skimmed or skimmed milk. Three or four cups of ground coffee. Unlimited green/black/white tea, camomile tea and mineral water. Freshly squeezed apple juice (and other freshly squeezed juices)**

- **Supplements: see page 113**

Over the next few days I describe some moderately advanced complementary therapies. When you find a therapy that appeals to you, research all the ways you can use it in your daily life.

Daily breathing exercise

From today onward I'd like you to do one "set" of breathing (see below) three times per day. I'd also like you to keep a daily record of your pulse rate, CP and inhaler use (copy and use the chart below). This will allow you to assess easily your progress on day fourteen of the program. A set consists of the following actions.

One set of breathing

1 Breathe gently and normally for five minutes.

2 Record your pulse rate and your CP.

3 Take shallow breaths for 10 minutes.

4 Breathe gently and normally for three minutes.

5 Record your pulse rate and your CP.

Magnetic therapy

Buy a magnetic chain to wear around your neck. Magnetic therapy boosts circulation, promotes healing and reduces pain, and you may find that it benefits your asthma. Magnetic jewelry is widely available in chemists, healthfood shops and online. The Energetix range (www.energetix.tv) is available in most countries and includes many items designed for men, too.

Monitoring your progress on the Buteyko method

date	control pause (seconds)	pulse rate	reliever inhaler usage (puffs)

day nine

Daily menu

- **Breakfast: Low-Sulfite Muesli (see page 132) with chopped fruit**

- **Morning snack: a large apple**

- **Lunch: bowl of chopped avocado, freshly cooked non-sulfited prawns and mixed salad leaves drizzled with olive oil and fresh lemon juice, and sprinkled with seeds. Bread roll**

- **Afternoon snack: handful of Brazil nuts**

- **Dinner: halibut steak baked with fresh lemon juice, olive oil, garlic and chopped herbs. Baked potato. Roast tomatoes, red peppers and courgettes. Baked apple drizzled with honey and chopped walnuts**

- **Drinks: 570ml/20fl oz/scant 2¹/₃ cups semi-skimmed or skimmed milk. Three or four cups of ground coffee. Unlimited green/black/white tea, camomile tea and mineral water. Freshly squeezed apple juice (and other freshly squeezed juices)**

- **Supplements: see page 113**

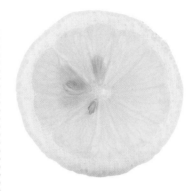

Whenever you feel an asthma attack coming on, the Buteyko method for dealing with it is as follows. Do a control pause (CP) test, then practise reduced breathing for three to five minutes, then do a CP test, followed by normal, gentle breathing. If this doesn't improve your symptoms, use your reliever inhaler.

Daily breathing exercise

Do one set of breathing three times today (see day eight). Remember to record your pulse rate, CP and inhaler use.

Homeopathy

Although it's best to consult a homeopath for individual advice, there are some remedies you can try by yourself – consult the chart on page 30 and select the remedy that most accurately describes your situation. You may previously have taken a remedy at the 6c potency during the gentle program. Now I'd like you take it in a potency of 12c, twice a day for five days. Alternatively, if you saw a homeopath at the end of the gentle program, keep taking those remedies.

Sleep in silk

Invest in silk bedding, or even a silk-filled duvet for the ultimate, anti-allergy luxury. As well as being light, soft and sensual, silk is hypoallergenic, breathable and chemical-free. Silk thread is made up of 18 amino acids that are also found in the human body, so reactions against it are rare. And, importantly, dust mites do not colonize it, so a silk-filled duvet remains mite-free – unlike feather-filled and synthetic duvets, which can harbour up to 20,000 live house dust mites. Wash non-silk duvets at 60°C, every three months, to limit their colonization with mites.

the moderate program day ten

Daily menu

- **Breakfast: smoothie made by whizzing a banana, some raspberries, some low-fat bio yogurt and a handful of flaked almonds in a food processor**

- **Morning snack: a large apple**

- **Lunch: home-made vegetable soup (see page 112), such as French onion. Bread roll**

- **Afternoon snack: handful of walnuts**

- **Dinner: Roasted Lemony Chicken with Tarragon (see page 136) with Sage & Onion Stuffing (see page 136). Carrots. Broccoli. Boiled sweet potatoes. Chopped oranges and strawberries sprinkled with chopped mint**

- **Drinks: 570ml/20fl oz/scant 2¹/₃ cups semi-skimmed or skimmed milk. Three or four cups of ground coffee. Unlimited green/black/white tea, camomile tea and mineral water. Freshly squeezed apple juice (and other freshly squeezed juices)**

- **Supplements: see page 113**

Daily breathing exercise

Do your usual set of breathing three times (see day eight). Buteyko also uses a technique called the extended pause (see below), which involves holding your breath long enough for your carbon dioxide level to start building up – this is thought to dilate your airways.

Extended pause

1 Begin as you would for the CP (see day four) but, this time, when you first feel the need to breathe in, hold your breath for a few seconds longer to get a stronger feeling of air hunger.
2 Now breathe in gently, then let out a little bit of air so your lungs don't feel full, or empty, but just comfortable.
3 Pinch your nostrils closed and hold your breath with your mouth closed until you feel the desire to breathe in. This is your control pause time. Now, instead of inhaling, hold your breath for two seconds longer, then breathe in gently through your nose.
4 With practice, you can build up to holding your breath five to 10 seconds longer than your CP time – but hold your breath only to a level that allows you to resume normal, gentle breathing. You shouldn't need to gasp for air.

Herbalism

Today, I'd like you to add a herbal medicine to your complementary health regime. The remedy I've selected is *Boswellia serrata* (frankincense) – an anti-inflammatory resin that can significantly improve asthma symptoms (see page 26). Select a product supplying around 200mg and take it twice a day.

Alternatively, if your asthma is triggered by hayfever, try taking herbal supplements containing butterbur (*Petasites hybridus*). Research shows this is as effective at treating hayfever symptoms as an over-the-counter antihistamine (for example, cetirizine), but without the side-effect of drowsiness. Choose standardized butterbur products, containing a known amount of the active ingredient petasin, and that are certified free of pyrrolizidine alkaloids.

day eleven

Daily menu

- **Breakfast: toast made with Low-Sulfite Soda Bread (see page 132). Low-Sulfite Old-English Marmalade (see page 133)**

- **Morning snack: a large apple**

- **Lunch: cold roast chicken. Minted Pea, Cucumber and Spring Onion Salad (see page 135). Bowl of mixed salad leaves drizzled with olive oil and fresh lemon juice, and sprinkled with seeds. Bread roll**

- **Afternoon snack: handful of Brazil nuts**

- **Dinner: Pasta with Creamy Walnut and Coriander Pesto (see page 136). Summer Pudding (see page 141)**

- **Drinks: 570ml/20fl oz/scant 2$^1/_3$ cups semi-skimmed or skimmed milk. Three to four cups of ground coffee. Unlimited green/black/white tea, camomile tea and mineral water. Freshly squeezed apple juice (and other freshly squeezed juices)**

- **Supplements: see page 113**

Instead of Brazil nuts you can eat macadamia nuts for your afternoon snack. Macadamia nut oil contains more than 80 percent monounsaturated fat – the highest of any oil, including olive oil. Macadamias are also a good source of fibre, protein, calcium and antioxidants. Macadamia and other nut butters make a great, nutritious snack spread on oatcakes or crisp breads. Choose organic versions that don't contain sulfite preservatives.

Daily breathing exercise

Do one set of breathing, three times today, as you did on day eight. Also repeat the extended pause technique you learned yesterday, and hold your breath for slightly longer – three seconds beyond your control pause time. Your aim is to develop a feeling of slight air hunger that is sustained over a short period. Do this two or three times every day, until your control pause lengthens and your asthma improves.

Meditation

This meditation technique helps to reduce stress-related asthma attacks. It involves repeating a word or phrase – known as a mantra – in your mind.

Reciting a mantra

1. Select a word, such as "calm", to say to yourself as you breathe out. Alternatively, choose a sound such as "shhhh" or "om".
2. Close your eyes and sit quietly, gently breathing in and out through your nose.
3. When you feel ready start to say your mantra silently on each exhalation in a rhythmic and relaxed way.
4. Do this for five minutes today, and whenever you are stressed.

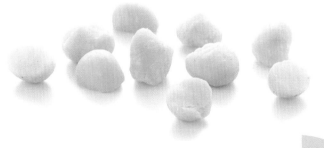

the moderate program
day twelve

Daily menu

- Breakfast: Low-Sulfite Muesli (see page 132) with chopped fruit

- Morning snack: a large apple

- Lunch: home-made chicken and vegetable soup (see page 112). Bread roll

- Afternoon snack: handful of walnuts

- Dinner: Grilled Tuna with Lemon and Mint Bulgur Wheat Salad (see page 138). Grilled red grapefruit drizzled with honey

- Drinks: 570ml/20fl oz/scant 2^1/$_3$ cups semi-skimmed or skimmed milk. Three or four cups of ground coffee. Unlimited green/black/white tea, camomile tea and mineral water. Freshly squeezed apple juice (and other freshly squeezed juices)

- Supplements: see page 113

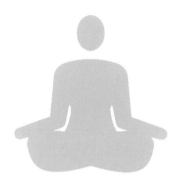

Daily breathing exercise

Do one set of breathing three times today (see day eight). Also, from now on, try to be aware of your breathing pattern at all times. Do spot checks on your breathing at intervals throughout the day. If you are breathing through your mouth, stop and breathe through your nose. If you're taking large, deep breaths, make a conscious effort to take in a little less air with each breath so that you develop a slight hunger for air.

Visualization

Another technique that can help asthma is visualization.

Sea breeze

1 Sit quietly with your eyes closed while breathing in and out gently through your nose.

2 Imagine yourself by the ocean, breathing in the cool, cleansing ocean breeze. Feel the sea spray against your skin.

3 As you inhale the sea air, visualize your airways dilating, and becoming more and more open, relaxed and elastic. As each breath leaves your body, visualize it as grey smoke transporting toxins and inflammation away.

4 Do this for five minutes today and whenever your chest starts to feel tight.

Boost immunity with garlic

A traditional daily Ayurvedic remedy for asthma involves heating 10 cloves of fresh garlic in 6tbsp (more if necessary) of milk for 20 minutes. Strain the milk and drink it. Garlic has powerful antiseptic, antiviral and anti-inflammatory properties that can reduce hayfever symptoms, as well as reduce your susceptibility to respiratory infections that can trigger asthma.

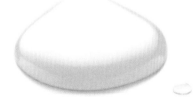

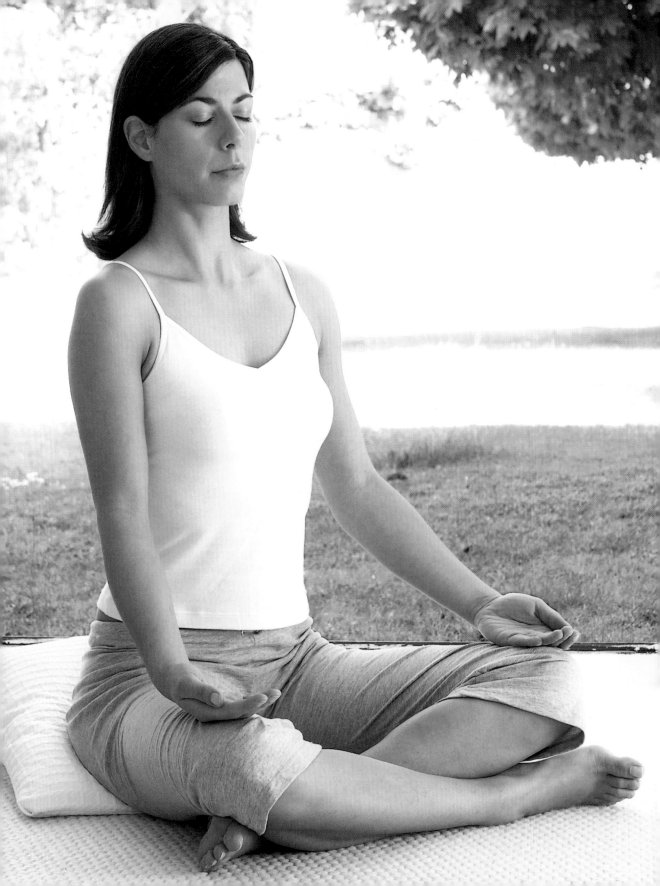

the moderate program day thirteen

Daily menu

- **Breakfast: porridge made with rolled oats, and sprinkled with chopped banana and mixed nuts**

- **Morning snack: a large apple**

- **Lunch: Salmon Ceviche with Lime and Coriander (see page 134). Bowl of mixed salad leaves drizzled with olive oil and fresh lemon juice, and sprinkled with seeds. Bread roll**

- **Afternoon snack: handful of Brazil nuts**

- **Dinner: cubes of lamb and chunks of onion, tomato and red pepper threaded onto skewers, brushed with olive oil and grilled. Brown rice. Courgettes. Corn-on-the-cob. Poached Apricots with Honey (see page 140)**

- **Drinks: 570ml/20fl oz/scant 2¹/₃ cups semi-skimmed or skimmed milk. Three or four cups of ground coffee. Unlimited green/black/white tea, camomile tea and mineral water. Freshly squeezed apple juice (and other freshly squeezed juices)**

- **Supplements: see page 113**

Today's menu includes fresh, poached apricots. Avoid preserved, dried or ready-to-eat semi-dried apricots unless they're organic without added sulfites. You can recognize sulfited apricots by their bright orange colour; those that are non-sulfited turn dull brown.

Daily breathing exercise

By now, you should be able to do around eight to 10 sets of breathing (as described on day eight) per day. Start to integrate reduced breathing into your daily life. Your ultimate aim is to perform reduced breathing (known as hypoventilation) all day every day, so that it's reflexive.

Acupressure

I describe some acupressure points to treat asthma on page 36. The most important of these is Stomach 16, also called Ying Chuang or "Stop Asthma" – you're going to stimulate this today.

Stimulating Stomach 16

1 Locate the acupoint on the front of your chest on each side, just below your third rib, and directly above your nipple.

2 Press on both sides lightly with your index fingers, while breathing slowly through your nose.

3 Gradually increase the pressure of your fingers until the points feel tender, then slowly decrease the pressure. Do this sequentially for five minutes, twice a day, morning and evening, from now on.

Foods that contain histamine

Some people with asthma will benefit from avoiding foods that contain histamine – it is found in improperly cleaned and refrigerated scromboid fish (especially tuna), fermented foods (for example, sauerkraut), cheese, tomato, spinach, aubergine, berries and citrus fruits. If the moderate program hasn't made a significant impact on your asthma symptoms, it may be worth avoiding these foods for the next two weeks. If this doesn't help, move on to the full-strength program.

day fourteen

Daily menu

- **Breakfast: toast made with Low-Sulfite Soda Bread (see page 132). Low-Sulfite Raspberry Jam (see page 133)**

- **Morning snack: a large apple**

- **Lunch: Spinach and Rice Soup (see page 134). Bread roll**

- **Afternoon snack: handful of walnuts**

- **Dinner: Tagliatelle with Herby Lemon and Walnut butter (see page 138). Cottage cheese mixed with freshly chopped pears, walnuts and blueberries**

- **Drinks: 570ml/20fl oz/scant $2^1/_3$ cups semi-skimmed or skimmed milk. Three or four cups of ground coffee. Unlimited green/black/white tea, camomile tea and mineral water. Freshly squeezed apple juice (and other freshly squeezed juices)**

- **Supplements: see page 113**

Daily breathing exercise

By now, your control pause (CP) should have improved by a further one or two seconds over your result on day seven of this program (check your chart). Continue to measure your CP once a day – if it starts to reduce, spend more time on your daily shallow breathing exercises.

Consulting a Buteyko practitioner

After two weeks you should now be aware of a significant improvement in your asthma symptoms. It's time to consult another complementary therapist and, having introduced you to several Buteyko practices during this program, I suggest you now visit a Buteyko practitioner to check you are doing the exercises correctly, and to learn more advanced techniques, such as the maximum pause. The Buteyko Institute Method is usually offered as a series of five sessions, each lasting 90 minutes, with further review sessions scheduled in as necessary. Most courses involve small groups, but some practitioners give one-to-one tuition if you prefer. A teacher will guide you through the Buteyko breathing exercises, most of which are carried out while sitting comfortably in a chair. To find a Buteyko practitioner, check the resources section on page 174.

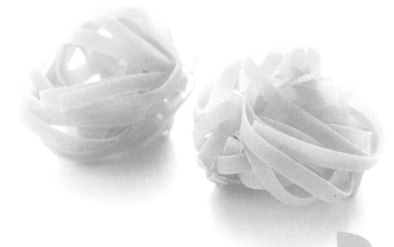

continuing the moderate program

Well done – you have followed the moderate program for two weeks. Now you need to assess whether or not reducing your exposure to dietary sulfites has helped your asthma symptoms. If you haven't noticed a significant improvement in your symptoms, I suggest you follow the gentle program if you haven't already done so. If you have previously followed the gentle program, please move on to the full-strength program to find out whether or not your asthma is improved by reducing your exposure to dietary salicylates.

If you *have* noticed a significant improvement in your asthma, you need to confirm whether or not your asthma is triggered by sulfites, or whether your improvement is linked to practising the Buteyko exercises. If you feel comfortable doing so, try eating foods containing sulfites for one day to see if your symptoms worsen. If they do, then continue to minimize your exposure to foods containing high amounts of these in the future. If your asthma does not worsen again, then slowly start to re-introduce sulfite-containing foods to your diet while continuing with the Buteyko exercises.

Your long-term diet

The moderate program offers a healthy way to eat that also reduces your exposure to dietary sulfites. If you're sensitive to sulfites, you need to be aware of all the foods that contain them – they may be added to foods or naturally present. Look at the chart on page 47. When you are buying ready-made foods always check the food labels. If sulfites have been added, they may be referred to as an E number anywhere between E220 and E228. The words "sulfur dioxide" or "sodium bisulfite" also mean that sulfites are present in a food. Over-the-counter or prescribed medicines may also contain sulfites, so check with a pharmacist or doctor before taking a medicine. If you take a drug or eat a food containing sulfites, you risk developing symptoms such as those described on page 46, as well as experiencing an asthma attack.

In your daily diet, concentrate on eating at least four or five servings of salad and vegetables (not including potatoes) and two or three servings of fruit as snacks. Always select organic products as these should not contain any food additives or preservatives.

Recipes Explore recipes containing sulfite-free foods, especially fish-based and vegetarian recipes – you will find some recipe suggestions at

Increase your level of exercise
When you can comfortably manage 30 minutes a day of aerobic exercise, try gradually to increase this. Exercise is not only important for your long-term cardiovascular health, it can also help you to gain and maintain a healthy weight. Brisk walking, cycling, swimming, dancing, gardening, bowling and golf are great forms of exercise and are also beneficial for the health of your lungs.

www.naturalhealthguru.co.uk and you can post your own favourites there, too, for other followers of the moderate program to try. If this style of eating works for you, and your asthma symptoms are well controlled, aim to follow its principles for the rest of your life.

Your long-term supplement regime

Continue to take the recommended supplements for the moderate program (see page 113) long-term. Research supports their use at this moderately high level for significant beneficial effects on lung function and asthma symptoms. If, up until now, you have taken only the supplements in the desirable list, you may wish to add in one or more of the supplements in the optional list for extra benefit. Alternatively, if your asthma symptoms are well controlled, you may wish to reduce the dose of your supplements back down to the levels suggested in the gentle program. This stepping down of your supplements is similar in principle to the stepping down of the asthma treatments in your personal asthma management plan (see pages 20–21). If you feel the higher dose suits you better, you can always step the supplement doses back up to those suggested in the moderate program – or even increase them to those I suggest in the full-strength program. If you do step down or step up your supplement doses, please continue to take the vitamin-B12 supplement, as this is particularly aimed at people with a sulfite intolerance.

Your exercise routine

Having followed the breath control exercises based on the Buteyko method, you should already have noticed an improvement in your lung function. Continue with these exercises or, if you prefer, move on to the yoga-based, pranayama exercises I have included in the full-strength program. You don't have to follow the full-strength menu plans – just substitute your Buteyko exercises for pranayama exercises. Alternatively, you can go back to using the simpler breathing exercises included in the gentle program. Once you've tried all the exercises, you'll know which ones work best for you, and then you can stick to them.

Aim to fit in at least 30 minutes of brisk exercise during most days, too. You don't have to complete your exercise all in one go – two daily sessions of 15 minutes or three daily sessions of 10 minutes are just as good for your long-term health as one longer one. Find a form of exercise that appeals to you – the more you enjoy your chosen activity, the more motivated you will be to keep it up. If exercise triggers your asthma, follow the tips I've given on pages 68–69 to help overcome this problem.

Your therapy program

The moderate program has shown you how to use reflexology to benefit your breathing, and introduced you to several other complementary techniques, including magnetic therapy, homeopathy, herbal medicine, meditation and visualization. Continue to use the therapies you have found most beneficial, and continue to consult the reflexologist and Buteyko practitioner if you found their advice helpful.

Monitoring your asthma

Continue to record your peak flow measurements on a chart (see page 77). This gives you early warning if your asthma control is starting to deteriorate. Ideally, you want to keep your peak flow readings within 20 percent of your personal best reading (see pages 16–17). If your readings go below 20 percent of your personal best, make an appointment to see your doctor or asthma nurse. Also check to see if you have inadvertently included a source of sulfites in your diet that might be adversely affecting your asthma control.

breakfast recipes

low-sulfite soda bread

. . . .

makes 1 loaf

450g/1lb/3½ cups unbleached white
flour
1 tsp salt
1 tsp bicarbonate of soda
350–400ml/12–14fl oz/scant 1½–scant
1²⁄₃ cups sour milk or butter milk

1   Preheat the oven to
230°C/450°F/Gas 8. Sift the dry
ingredients into a bowl. Make
a well in the middle and pour
in most of the milk. Mix in the
flour from the sides, adding
more milk if necessary to make
a soft dough that is not too wet
and sticky.

2   Put the dough on a floured
surface and pat it into a round
about 2.5cm/1in thick. Cut a
cross in the surface. Transfer
to a baking sheet and bake for
15 minutes, then turn down
the oven to 200°C/400°F/Gas
6 for a further 30 minutes or
until cooked. Tap the base of
the bread – it will sound hollow
when it is cooked.

low-sulfite muesli

. . . .

serves 4

1 handful rolled oats
1 handful mixed muesli cereals, such
as toasted wheat flakes, rye flakes,
barley flakes, bran flakes
1 handful mixed, chopped nuts, such
as walnuts, Brazil nuts and flaked
almonds
1 handful mixed seeds, such as
sunflower, pumpkin and sesame
seeds
Semi-skimmed milk, to serve
Dried apricots, dates or figs without
sulfites, to serve (optional)

1   Mix all the ingredients together
and divide into 4 bowls.

2   Serve with milk and dried fruit.

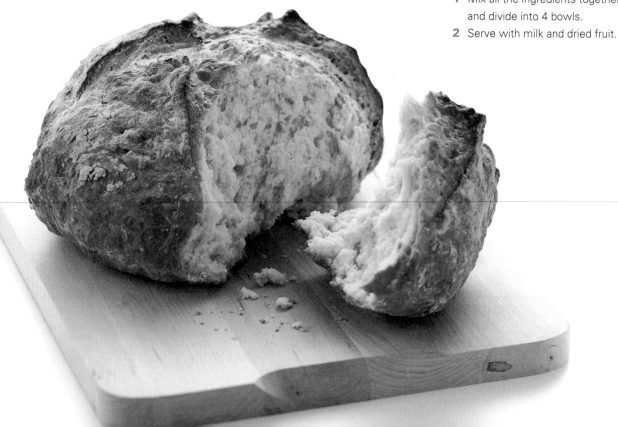

low-sulfite raspberry jam

makes 3 jars

700g/1lb 9oz/3 cups caster sugar
900g/2lb raspberries

1 Preheat the oven to 180°C/350°F/Gas 4. Wash and dry 3 x 450g/1lb jam jars and lids, then sterilize them in the hot oven for 15 minutes.

2 Put the sugar in an ovenproof bowl and heat in the oven for 5–10 minutes. Meanwhile, put the raspberries in a stainless steel pan and heat gently for 4 minutes until the juice begins to run.

3 Add the hot sugar and stir over gentle heat until fully dissolved. Bring to the boil and simmer gently for 5 minutes, stirring frequently. Put a teaspoon of jam on a cold plate and press with a finger when cool. If the surface wrinkles, the jam is set.

4 Remove from the heat, skim and pour into the jam jars. Cover with the lids, then label and store in a cool dry place.

low-sulfite old-english marmalade

makes 10 jars

1.5kg/3lb 5oz oranges
2.5kg/5lb 8oz/11 cups caster sugar

1 Preheat the oven to 180°C/350°F/Gas 4. Wash and dry 10 x 450g/1lb jam jars and lids, then sterilize them in the hot oven for 15 minutes.

2 Remove and shred the peel of the oranges and put it in a large bowl. Cut the orange flesh into small pieces, removing and retaining the pips.

3 Add the chopped orange flesh to the peel and cover with 3.5l/122fl oz/3¾ quarts water. Leave to marinate for 12 hours, or overnight.

4 Put the pips in a small pan, adding just enough water to cover them. Bring to the boil and then take off the heat. Leave to infuse for 12 hours or overnight.

5 Extract the pips from the jelly that has formed around them.

6 Put the jelly in a large pan with the orange peel mixture and bring to the boil. Simmer gently for 1½–2 hours until the peel is soft.

7 Gradually add the sugar and boil until the setting point is reached. Remove from the heat, skim and pour into the jam jars. Cover with the sterilized lids. Label and store in a cool dry place.

scrambled eggs with red pepper and tomato

serves 4

1 tbsp olive oil
2 garlic cloves, crushed
1 red pepper, deseeded and cut into strips
2 large tomatoes, chopped
6 large eggs, beaten
1 handful parsley, chopped
Freshly ground black pepper

1 Lightly brush the base of a pan with the oil. Fry the garlic, red pepper and tomatoes until soft.

2 Add the eggs and cook 2–3 minutes, stirring continuously until scrambled. Season well with black pepper, sprinkle parsley on top and serve.

left: low-sulfite soda bread

lunch recipes

avocado dip

serves 4

1 handful watercress, chopped
A few coriander leaves, chopped
1 tsp ground coriander
1 green chilli, deseeded and finely
    chopped
Juice and zest of 1 unwaxed lime
2 avocados, peeled, stoned and mashed
150ml/5fl oz/^{2}/$_3$ cup low-fat bio yogurt
2 spring onions, finely chopped
Freshly ground black pepper
Crackers or bread, to serve

1 Put the watercress, coriander
   leaves, ground coriander and
   chilli in a food processor with
   the lime juice and zest and
   blend until finely chopped.
2 Combine the watercress
   mixture with the avocado flesh.
   Add the yogurt and spring
   onions. Season with black
   pepper, stir well, then cover
   and chill. Serve with crackers
   or bread.

crab and orange salad

serves 4

400g/14oz fresh crab meat
1 handful parsley, chopped, to serve

For the dressing:
Juice and zest of 2 unwaxed oranges
4 tbsp extra virgin olive oil
Freshly ground black pepper

1 Whisk together the orange
   juice, zest, olive oil and plenty
   of black pepper to make the
   dressing.
2 Put the crab meat in a small
   bowl and moisten with some of
   the dressing.
3 Put a small entrée-preparation
   ring on a serving plate and
   spoon in a quarter of the crab
   meat. Sprinkle with some of
   the parsley and a little of the
   dressing. Carefully remove
   the ring to leave a neat round
   of crab. Repeat to make four
   rounds, then serve.

salmon ceviche with lime and coriander

serves 4

225g/8oz ultra-fresh, sushi-grade raw
    salmon fillet, chopped
4 handfuls mixed salad leaves
½ cucumber, peeled and chopped
4 spring onions, chopped

For the marinade:
Juice and zest of 4 unwaxed limes
4 tbsp extra virgin olive oil
2 tomatoes, skinned and chopped
1 green chilli, deseeded and finely
    chopped
1 handful coriander leaves, finely
    chopped
2 tsp caster sugar
Freshly ground black pepper

1 Combine the marinade
   ingredients in a non-metallic
   bowl and season well with
   black pepper.
2 Add the salmon and mix well.
   Cover and chill for 3 hours,
   stirring occasionally, until the
   salmon is pink and opaque.
3 Put the salmon on the salad
   leaves, sprinkle with the
   cucumber and spring onions
   and serve.

spinach and rice soup

serves 4

1 onion, finely chopped
2 garlic cloves, crushed
4 thyme sprigs
2 rosemary sprigs
2 tsp coriander seeds, ground
4 tbsp olive oil
125g/4½oz/heaped ½ cup risotto
   (Arborio) rice
1.1l/38½fl oz/4½ cup home-made
   vegetable stock (see page 112)
225g/8oz baby leaf spinach, chopped
Juice and zest of 1 small unwaxed
   lemon
Freshly ground black pepper

1 Sauté the onion, garlic, thyme,
   rosemary and coriander seeds
   in the olive oil for 5 minutes.
   Add the rice and cook, stirring,
   for 1 minute. Add the stock and
   bring to the boil. Simmer gently
   for 20 minutes until the rice
   is tender.
2 Stir the spinach, lemon juice
   and zest into the soup and cook
   for 2 minutes. Season well with
   black pepper, then serve.

*minted pea, cucumber and
spring onion salad*

sulfite-free coleslaw

serves 4

1 green apple, peeled
Juice and zest of 2 unwaxed lemons
½ small white cabbage, shredded
2 carrots, grated
1 red onion, thinly sliced
1 handful chopped herbs, such as dill
   or parsley
150ml/5fl oz/²/₃ cup low-fat bio yogurt
Freshly ground black pepper

1 Grate the apple and mix with
   the lemon juice and zest.
2 Combine the apple mixture
   with the remaining ingredients.
   Season well with black pepper.

minted pea, cucumber and spring onion salad

serves 4

450g/1lb/3 cups shelled garden peas
½ cucumber, peeled and chopped
4 spring onions, chopped
150ml/5fl oz/²/₃ cup low-fat crème
   fraîche
1 handful mint, chopped
Freshly ground black pepper

1 Cook the peas in boiling water
   for 5 minutes. Drain and leave
   to cool.
2 Combine all the ingredients in
   a bowl, season well with black
   pepper and serve.

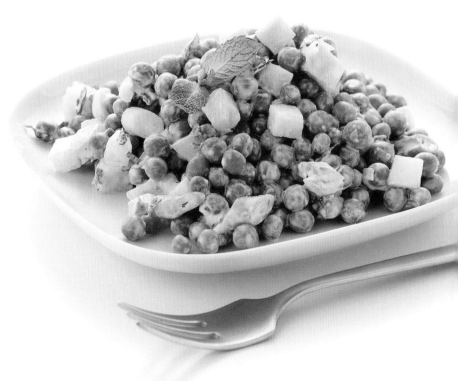

dinner recipes

roasted lemony chicken with tarragon

serves 4

1 chicken
1 handful tarragon, chopped
55g/2oz butter
1 unwaxed lemon, halved
Freshly ground black pepper
1 recipe quantity Sage and Onion
   Stuffing (see right)

1 Preheat the oven to
   200°C/400°F/Gas 6. Make
   small cuts in the skin on the
   chicken breasts and tuck in the
   tarragon. Rub the top of the
   chicken with the butter.
2 Squeeze the lemon over the
   chicken and put the lemon
   halves inside the chicken.
3 Season well with black pepper
   and roast for 1½–2 hours,
   depending on weight. Pierce a
   chicken thigh with a skewer to
   check it is cooked – the juices
   should run clear. Serve with
   the stuffing.

sage and onion stuffing

serves 4

30g/1oz butter
1 large onion, chopped
1 handful sage, chopped
4 slices wholemeal bread, finely
   chopped
1 egg
Freshly ground black pepper
1 recipe quantity Roasted Lemony
   Chicken with Tarragon (see left)

1 Preheat the oven to
   200°C/400°F/Gas 6. Put the
   butter in a pan and melt over
   a low heat. Sauté the onion
   until soft. Remove from the
   heat and add the sage and the
   bread. Season well with black
   pepper and mix.
2 Break the egg over the mixture
   and combine thoroughly. Put
   the mixture in an ovenproof
   dish and bake during the last
   30 minutes of the chicken's
   cooking time (see left).

pasta with creamy walnut and coriander pesto

serves 4

4 tbsp walnut oil
1 handful walnuts, crushed
2 garlic cloves, crushed
1 handful coriander leaves, chopped
1 handful parsley, chopped
1 tsp coriander seeds, crushed
60g/2oz/¼ cup mascarpone cheese
   (or crème fraîche)
450g/1lb fresh pasta
Freshly ground black pepper

1 Blend or pound the oil, nuts,
   garlic, herbs and spices into a
   smooth paste.
2 Stir in the mascarpone and
   season with black pepper.
3 Cook the pasta in plenty of
   boiling water, according to the
   packet instructions, until al
   dente. Drain but leave moist
   so the sauce will coat the
   pasta well.
4 Combine the pasta and
   sauce and toss well.
   Serve immediately.

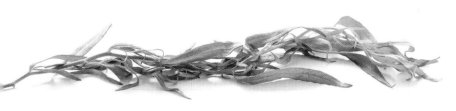

duck à l'orange

serves 4

4 duck breasts
1 tsp ground allspice
1 tbsp olive oil
Juice and zest of 2 unwaxed oranges
400ml/14fl oz/1²/₃ cups chicken stock
   (made by boiling bones and
   vegetables; see page 112)
Freshly ground black pepper

1 Make 3–4 cuts in the duck skin
   and rub with the allspice and
   black pepper.
2 Fry the duck breasts in the
   olive oil over medium heat
   for 6–8 minutes on each side,
   depending on size and how
   well done you like them.
   Remove from the pan, slice
   and cover with foil.
3 To make the sauce, pour off
   most of the fat in the pan, then
   add the orange juice, zest and
   stock. Bring to the boil and
   simmer for 5 minutes until the
   liquid has reduced by half.
4 Pour the sauce over the duck
   slices, season with black
   pepper and serve.

red rice pilaf

serves 4

250g/9oz/1¼ cups Camargue red rice
1 large onion, finely chopped
55g/2oz butter
1 handful parsley, chopped
Freshly ground black pepper

1 Cook the rice according to the
   packet instructions and drain.
2 Sauté the onion in the butter.
   Stir in the rice and parsley and
   season well with black pepper.

beef tenderloin with brown mushrooms and potatoes

serves 4

1.3kg/3lb beef tenderloin joint
450g/1lb brown mushrooms, quartered
8 potatoes, peeled and sliced
30g/1oz butter
Freshly ground black pepper

1 Preheat the oven to
   180°C/350°F/Gas 4. Put all the
   ingredients and 125ml/4fl oz/½
   cup water in a roasting tin.

2 Season well with black pepper.
   Bake for 35 minutes, or longer
   if you prefer your beef well
   done, basting halfway through,
   then serve.

spicy mackerel

serves 4

4 small mackerel fillets
Freshly ground black pepper

For the marinade:
4 tbsp olive oil
Juice and zest of 1 unwaxed lemon
1 red chilli, deseeded and finely
   chopped
3 garlic cloves, crushed
1 tsp ground coriander
1 tsp ground cumin
1 handful coriander, chopped

1 Put all the marinade ingredients
   in a bowl and mix well.
2 Put the mackerel fillets in a
   shallow dish, skin-side down,
   and cover with the marinade.
   Season well with black pepper
   and leave for 1 hour.
3 Grill the fish for 8–10 minutes
   until cooked and crisp,
   then serve.

grilled tuna with lemon and mint bulgur wheat salad

serves 4

125g/4½oz/¾ cup bulgur wheat, rinsed
2 garlic cloves, crushed
Juice and zest of 2 unwaxed lemons
4 tbsp olive oil
4 ultra-fresh, sushi-grade tuna steaks
4 spring onions, finely chopped
12 cherry tomatoes, halved
1 handful mint, chopped
1 handful parsley, chopped
Freshly ground black pepper

1 Put the bulgur wheat in a pan, cover with water and bring to the boil. Simmer for 4 minutes, then remove from the heat and leave to stand for 15 minutes.
2 Combine the garlic, half the lemon juice and zest, and the olive oil. Season well with black pepper. Use some of the mixture to coat the tuna steaks.
3 Grill the steaks for 2–3 minutes on each side depending on their thickness. Mix the bulgur wheat with the remaining lemon juice and zest, the spring onions, tomatoes, mint and parsley. Season with black pepper. Put the tuna on a bed of bulgur wheat and serve.

tagliatelle with herby lemon and walnut butter

serves 4

55g/2oz butter
85g/3oz/²/₃ cup walnuts, crushed
4 garlic cloves, crushed
Juice and zest of 2 unwaxed lemons
450g/1lb fresh or 225g/8oz dried tagliatelle
1 handful basil, chopped
1 handful parsley, chopped
2 tbsp single cream
Freshly ground black pepper

1 Melt the butter in a pan and add the walnuts and garlic. Cook for 30 seconds, then add the lemon zest and leave to cool.
2 Cook the tagliatelle according to the packet instructions. Drain well and stir in the walnut and garlic butter. Stir over a low heat for 3 minutes.
3 Add the herbs, lemon juice and single cream. Season well with black pepper and serve.

potato and smoked salmon pancakes

serves 4

225g/8oz potatoes, peeled
2 tbsp milk
4 tsp plain flour
2 small eggs, plus 2 egg whites
4 tsp double cream
15g/½oz butter
225g/8oz sulfite-free smoked salmon, chopped
1 handful parsley, chopped
Freshly ground black pepper

1 Boil the potatoes until tender. Drain well, then rub through a sieve into a bowl. Gently beat in the milk, then the flour, followed by the eggs and, finally, the cream to make a batter. Season with black pepper, cover and leave to stand for 30 minutes.
2 Melt a quarter of the butter in a frying pan over medium heat. When hot, put 4 separate dollops of batter in the pan, allowing room to spread. Cook for 30 seconds on each side, then put on a warm plate.
3 Put some smoked salmon on top of each pancake and keep warm in the oven. Add another quarter of the butter to the pan and repeat until the batter is used up. Sprinkle with the parsley and serve.

right: couscous with roast vegetables and tomato sauce

couscous with roast vegetables and tomato sauce

••••••••••••••••••••••••

serves 4

115g/4oz/²/3 cup couscous
1 red onion, thinly sliced
1 aubergine, halved and thinly sliced
   lengthways
1 courgette, thinly sliced lengthways
1 red pepper, deseeded and cut into
   strips
2 rosemary sprigs
4 garlic cloves, crushed
4 tbsp olive oil
Juice and zest of 1 unwaxed lemon
1 handful mint, chopped
1 handful parsley, chopped
1 handful coriander, chopped
Freshly ground black pepper

For the tomato sauce:
1 onion, finely chopped
2 tbsp olive oil

2 garlic cloves, crushed
12 plum tomatoes, skinned and
   chopped
Juice and zest of 1 unwaxed lemon
2 tsp sugar
Freshly ground black pepper

1 Preheat the oven to 200°C/400°F/Gas 6. Put the couscous in a large bowl, pour over 425ml/15fl oz/1¾ cups boiling water and leave to soak.

2 Place the vegetables and rosemary in a large roasting pan, sprinkle with the garlic, and drizzle with the olive oil and the lemon juice and zest. Roast for 30 minutes, turning occasionally.

3 Take the vegetables out of the oven, discard the rosemary

and mix the vegetables and chopped herbs with the couscous. Turn down the oven to 180°C/350°F/Gas 4. Pour the couscous mixture into 4 oiled 200ml/7fl oz/¾-cup moulds and pack down well. Cover with tin foil and bake for 15 minutes. Cool for 2 hours before unmoulding.

4 To make the tomato sauce, fry the onion in the olive oil until soft. Add the garlic and cook for a further 1 minute. Stir in the tomatoes, lemon juice, zest and sugar and simmer gently for 30 minutes, stirring occasionally. Season well with black pepper and serve with the couscous.

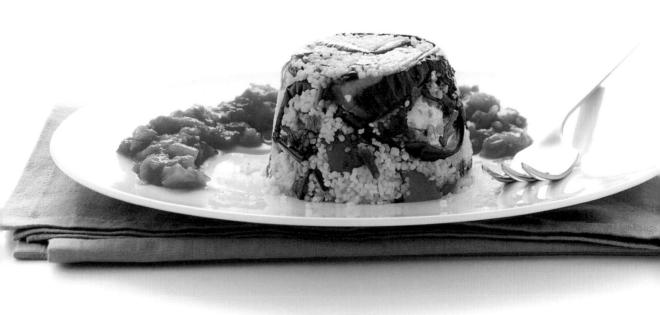

dessert recipes

almond-stuffed plums

serves 4

55g/2oz butter
55g/2oz/¼ cup caster sugar
55g/2oz/½ cup ground almonds
1 egg
12 plums
1 handful flaked almonds, toasted
Mascarpone cheese, to serve (optional)

1 Heat the oven to its highest setting. Mix the butter, sugar, ground almonds and egg together to form a paste.

2 Cut deep crosses in the top of each plum and remove the stones. Put a small lump of the almond paste into each plum and place in a roasting dish. Bake for 3–5 minutes until the juice starts to release.

3 Cool for 5 minutes, then sprinkle with the flaked almonds. Serve with mascarpone cheese, if using.

poached apricots with honey

serves 4

16 apricots, stoned and quartered
50g/1¾oz/¼ cup sugar
1 tbsp runny honey
Juice and zest of 1 unwaxed lime

1 Set a pan over a low heat, add the apricots, sugar and 150ml/5fl oz/ ²/₃ cup water and poach for 15 minutes.

2 Stir in the honey and the lime juice and zest and serve.

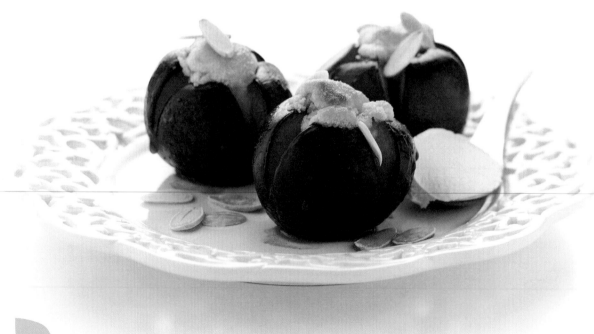

summer pudding

serves 4

12 slices of day-old white bread, crusts
    removed
800g/1lb 12oz mixed summer berries,
    such as raspberries, blueberries,
    blackcurrants, redcurrants and
    strawberries
50g/1¾oz/scant ¼ cup caster sugar

1 Line 4 small non-metallic
   moulds with bread, reserving
   enough to make a lid for each.
2 Put the fruit and sugar in a pan
   and heat gently for 3 minutes,
   stirring, until the sugar is
   dissolved and the fruit juices
   are starting to run.
3 Fill the bread-lined moulds with
   three quarters of the fruit. Put
   a bread lid on each and cover
   with clingfilm. Put a weight
   on each bread lid, and chill
   overnight.
4 Remove the moulds, sprinkle
   the remaining fruit over the
   puddings and serve.

apricot and walnut crumble

serves 4

16 apricots, stoned and quartered
2 tbsp caster sugar
55g/2oz/½ cup plain flour
55g/2oz/½ cup jumbo rolled oats
50g/1¾oz/¼ cup brown sugar
55g/2oz butter
30g/1oz/¼ cup walnuts, chopped

1 Preheat the oven to 190°C/
   375°F/Gas 5. Mix the apricots
   with the sugar and put the
   mixture in an ovenproof dish.
2 Mix the flour, oats and brown
   sugar in a mixing bowl, then
   rub in the butter to make the
   crumble topping. Stir in the
   chopped walnuts.
3 Spoon the crumble mix over
   the apricots and bake for
   30 minutes or until golden
   brown. Serve warm.

minted apples and berries

serves 4

Juice and zest of 2 unwaxed lemons
50g/1¾oz/scant ¼ cup caster sugar
600g/1lb 5oz cooking apples, peeled
    and chopped
150g/5½oz berries, such as blueberries,
    strawberries or raspberries
1 handful mint, chopped

1 Put the lemon juice and zest,
   half the sugar and the apples
   in a pan. Simmer gently for
   10 minutes until soft.
2 Put the apple in a food
   processor and blend until
   smooth. Cover and chill.
3 Put the berries and remaining
   sugar in a pan and heat gently
   until the juices start to run.
   Leave to cool.
4 Spoon alternate layers of
   apple and berries in 4 glasses,
   sprinkling each layer with a
   little mint, then serve.

left: almond-stuffed plums

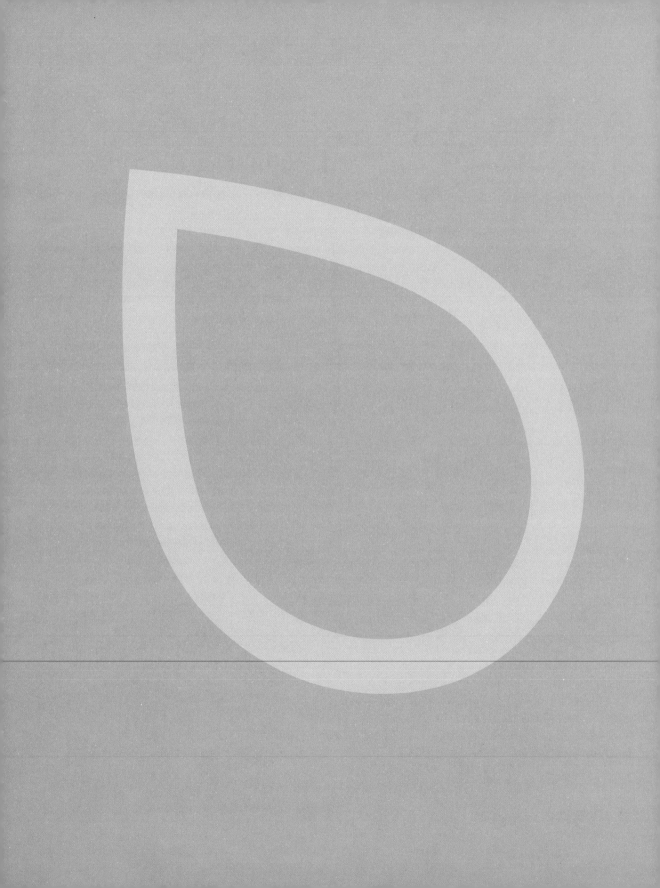

introducing the full-strength program

The full-strength program shows you how to follow a low-salicylate diet, how to incorporate yoga-based breathing exercises into your day, and how to perform some effective acupressure techniques to help improve your asthma. I recommend the full-strength program for people:

● Whose asthma has not significantly improved while following the antioxidant-rich diet of the gentle program.
● Whose asthma has not significantly improved while following the sulfite-elimination diet of the moderate program.
● Who know their asthma is sensitive to the drug aspirin.

I provide 14 daily plans that you can repeat so the program lasts for 28 days. Follow the program for at least one month before assessing its benefits. Once you feel comfortable with the diet and lifestyle changes involved, feel free to make your own adjustments that take into account your personal likes, dislikes and lifestyle, while still avoiding foods that exacerbate your asthma.

The full-strength diet

Over the next month your diet will exclude foods that have a significant salicylate content. As I described on pages 48–49, salicylates are natural, aspirin-like chemicals found in many fruit, vegetables, nuts, seeds, herbs and spices. Although they have a different chemical structure to aspirin, they cause the same build up of inflammatory chemicals in the lungs of those who are sensitive.

A typical Western diet provides 10–200mg salicylate a day (a typical aspirin tablet contains 300mg), which is enough to trigger asthma in sensitive people. One study found that the average amount of aspirin needed to produce a 15 percent decrease in peak flow in people with aspirin-sensitive asthma was 16.5mg aspirin. The most sensitive five percent of people reacted to a tiny dose of 0.8mg, while most (95 percent) reacted to a dose of 332.3mg. When it came to salicylates in food, the average amount needed to reduce peak flow by 15 percent was 15.3mg. The most sensitive five percent of people reacted to 2.6mg salicylate; and most people reacted to 89.9mg. This suggests that salicylates in food are as potent at triggering asthma as aspirin, if not more so.

It isn't viable to follow a salicylate-free diet as this wouldn't provide nutritional balance, but it's possible to reduce your intake. For example, some foods contain 4mg salicylates per 100g (3½oz), whereas my full-strength diet includes only foods that contain less than 0.5mg salicylates per 100g (3½oz) on average.

The full-strength diet is also tartrazine-free, as up to one in four people with salicylate-exacerbated asthma are also sensitive to this artificial yellow food colouring (see pages 50–51).

Fish in your diet A few people who are sensitive to aspirin may find that eating oily fish can worsen their

Shopping list

The following foods have a low salicylate content. Base your shopping lists around them.

drinks
camomile tea, carrot juice, grapefruit juice*, mineral water, rosehip tea, pineapple juice, wine

dairy products
butter (unsalted), buttermilk, cream (single and double), feta cheese, low-fat bio yogurt, low-fat cottage cheese, low-fat crème fraîche, mozzarella, Parmesan, plain uncoloured Cheddar cheese, quark, semi-skimmed/skimmed milk, sour cream

fruit
apples (Jonathan, Red Delicious and Golden Delicious only), bananas, figs (fresh only), grapefruit*, kiwi fruit, lemon, lime, lychees (canned), mango, papaya, passion fruit, pear (Williams only), plums, rhubarb
*Check for interactions between grapefruit and your medication

vegetables and salad stuff
baby sweetcorn, bamboo shoots (canned), beansprouts, beetroot, Brussels sprouts, carrots, cauliflower, celery, chickpeas, corn-on-the-cob, garden peas, green beans, green cabbage, kidney beans, leeks (including baby leeks), lentils, lettuce, lima beans, mangetout, mung beans, mushrooms (brown and oyster), onions, parsnips, pumpkin, red cabbage, shallots, soy beans, spinach (frozen), split peas (green and yellow), spring greens, spring onions, sweet potatoes, sweetcorn, tomatoes, turnips

nuts and seeds (unsalted)
Brazils, cashews, coconut (desiccated), hazelnuts, pecans, poppy seeds, sesame seeds, sunflower seeds, walnuts

herbs and spices
chives, coriander leaves, garlic, parsley, saffron

oils and condiments
extra virgin olive oil (for drizzling and dressings), olive oil (for cooking), malt vinegar, soy sauce

grains
breads (including pitta bread), breakfast cereals (except those containing cornmeal/cornflour), couscous, crackers, fresh/dried pasta (linguini, tagliatelle), pearl barley, rice (Basmati, brown, wild)

proteins
anchovies, bacon, cod, chicken, lamb, lemon sole, monkfish, mussels, omega-3 rich eggs, prosciutto, prawns, salmon, turkey

miscellaneous
brown sugar, cider (sweet and dry), fructose sugar, light tahini, peanut butter (but not fresh peanuts), rock salt

asthma symptoms. I have included a few fish dishes in the full-strength program, but if you find that these trigger your asthma, replace them with a vegetarian option, such as a stew made from low-salicylate vegetables. For a list of foods containing salicylates, see page 49.

Organic food – guidelines Although I usually advise people to eat organic food where possible, the full-strength program is the exception. If you're sensitive to salicylates it may be prudent to choose foods that don't have organic status. Researchers have found that organic plant foods tend to have a significantly higher salicylate content than non-organic products. This is because salicylates are protective substances produced by plants to safeguard them from disease, and which plants need in higher amounts when grown without artificial pesticides.

Select herbs and spices carefully You'll notice from the table on page 49 that a lot of spices and herbs are high-salicylate foods. It's therefore a good idea to avoid spicy food in general and to carefully check labels when buying pre-packaged foods. Ask for food to have minimal seasoning when eating out, too. It's also important to make your own stock/bouillon (see the recipe on page 172) and soups using low-salicylate plants and flavourings. This doesn't mean that your diet has to be bland. Select low-salicylate herbs such as coriander leaves, garlic, coconut and soy sauce to add flavour. Celery is virtually salicylate free and, although it's relatively tasteless on its own, it's well known as a food that brings out the flavour in other foods, especially meats. This is because it's packed full of chemicals that stimulate your savoury *umami* taste buds – receptors that were only recently identified as important for taste impact. Celery's volatile chemicals are especially good at accentuating the flavour of chicken.

Full-strength program supplements

The supplements I recommend in the full-strength program are similar to those in the previous programs but, where appropriate, at a higher, more therapeutic dose. Those in the recommended list of supplements are likely to have a beneficial effect on your asthma symptoms; those in the optional list have the potential to improve your symptoms even further. Read more about these supplements and their beneficial effects on pages 60–61. Avoid taking fish oil supplements if you know that fish oil exacerbates your asthma.

recommended daily supplements

- Vitamin C (1,500mg)
- Vitamin E (600mg)
- Vitamin B complex (50mg)
- Lycopene carotenoid complex (15mg)
- Magnesium (400mg)
- Selenium (200mcg)
- Omega-3 fish oils (3x1g fish oil capsules, each supplying 180mg EPA+120mg DHA; DHA-only blends are recommended during pregnancy)
- Pycnogenol (150mg)

optional daily supplements (these provide additional health benefits)

- Co-enzyme Q10 (90mg)
- Quercetin (500mg, three times a day before food)
- Bromelain (100mg, twice daily to enhance quercetin absorption)
- N-acetyl-l-cysteine (NAC) (100mg, three times a day)
- Reishi (1,500mg, or 500mg three times a day)
- Digestive enzymes (mixed; 4 capsules before meals)
- Probiotics (in the form of fermented milk drinks, bio yogurt or supplements)

The full-strength program exercise routine

Over the next two weeks, I'm going to explain some breathing exercises to help improve your breath control; they are based on yoga techniques known as pranayama. They're very different from the Buteyko exercises used in the moderate program, which encouraged you to take shallow breaths and to reduce the volume of air you inhale. In contrast, yogic exercises promote deep breathing to strengthen and relax your respiratory muscles. Try both the pranayama techniques and the Buteyko method, and adopt the technique that has the most positive impact on your breathing and your asthma symptoms.

In addition to daily breathing exercises, you should do at least 15 to 30 minutes of aerobic exercise once or twice a day. Aim to exercise for a longer duration as your fitness level improves. If you have problems with exercise-induced asthma, read the tips on pages 68–69 and use your reliever inhaler 15 minutes before starting your daily exercise regime.

Try to find new, interesting forms of exercise so you build variety into your exercise program – that way you won't get bored. As well as brisk walking, cycling and swimming, consider bowling, golf and similar activities that involve other people. That way, your social life improves as well as your health.

The full-strength program therapies

The complementary therapies I suggest for the full-strength program include acupressure, aromatherapy, naturopathy, homeopathy and meditation. I also recommend that you visit an acupuncturist and a nutritional therapist – you will need to book appointments with these therapists now, before you start the program (see pages 174–175).

the full-strength program day one

Daily menu

- **Breakfast: Prosciutto with Mango and Passion Fruit Relish (see page 164). Bread roll**

- **Morning snack: a large apple (Jonathan, Red Delicious or Golden Delicious only)**

- **Lunch: Mushroom Pâté (see page 167). Toast. Slices of tomato and red onion drizzled with olive oil and lemon juice and sprinkled with coriander leaves. Low-fat bio yogurt with allowed fruit and nuts**

- **Afternoon snack: handful of Brazil nuts**

- **Dinner: Linguini with a Saffron Prawn Sauce (see page 172). Frozen spinach, steamed. Tinned lychees (drained)**

- **Drinks: 570ml/20fl oz/scant 2$\frac{1}{3}$ cups semi-skimmed or skimmed milk. Camomile tea, rosehip tea and mineral water. One glass of grapefruit, pineapple or carrot juice**

- **Supplements: see page 145**

Daily breathing exercise

To start the full-strength breathing exercises, I'm going to show you a deceptively simple technique that can ease respiratory tension and help you relax.

Relaxing breath

1 Sit comfortably and place the tip of your tongue against the bony ridge behind your upper front teeth – keep it there for the duration of this exercise.

2 Breathe in through your nose as you silently count to four.

3 Hold your breath for a silent count of seven, then breathe

Ivy plants

Researchers have found that having a potted ivy plant growing in a room removes up to 80 percent of mould spores from your living space. The ivy absorbs substances from mould spores and stores them in its roots. If your asthma is trigged by mould, try having ivy plants in your home – it's a simple way to help control symptoms.

out through your mouth as you silently count to eight. Do this four times. Repeat this exercise whenever you feel tense or if you feel an asthma attack coming on.

Acupressure

During the first week of this program, I'd like you to use acupressure to complement the breathing program. Do today's exercise twice a day, morning and evening, for the rest of this week.

Stimulating Lung 11

1 Press on a point known as Lung 11, or Shao Shang, to reduce spasm in the airways. It's located beneath the outer corner of your thumb nail on both hands.

2 Start by stimulating the point on your right thumb, gradually increasing the pressure until it starts to feel uncomfortable, then gradually release the pressure.

3 Build up the pressure again, then slowly release. Repeat this a total of five times; then do the same on your left thumb.

day two

Daily menu

- **Breakfast: muesli with chopped banana (follow the recipe on page 132 but omit the almonds, dates and apricots)**

- **Morning snack: a large apple (Jonathan, Red Delicious or Golden Delicious only)**

- **Lunch: cottage cheese mixed with chopped Williams pear and cashew nuts. A bowl of lettuce mixed with chopped tomato, spring onion and celery, drizzled with olive oil and lemon juice and sprinkled with chives. Bread roll. Low-fat bio yogurt with allowed fruit and nuts**

- **Afternoon snack: handful of pecans**

- **Dinner: grilled salmon with garlic and lemon juice. Green beans. Carrots. Sweet potatoes. Banana and Walnut Bread (see page 173)**

- **Drinks: 570ml/20fl oz/scant 2¹⁄₃ cups semi-skimmed or skimmed milk. Camomile tea, rosehip tea and mineral water. One glass of grapefruit, pineapple or carrot juice**

- **Supplements: see page 145**

Today's afternoon snack is pecan nuts – they're a rich source of monounsaturated fatty acids and a good source of omega-3s, magnesium, zinc and selenium. They contain fewer salicylates than walnuts (see page 49).

Daily breathing exercise

Do today's exercise twice a day from now on, morning and evening, to start and end the day.

Upward stretch

1 Stand with your arms hanging loosely at your sides. Breathe in slowly through your nose to your fullest capacity.

2 As you breathe out through your mouth, move your arms out to the sides, palms up, then bring them up above your head.

3 Breathe in and bring your arms out to your sides and then over your head again. Feel your chest expand. Turn your palms to face down and, as you

slowly breathe out, push your palms down in front of you. Imagine you're pushing all the air out of your lungs. Repeat the whole exercise four times.

Acupressure

Stimulate Lung 11 as you did yesterday, then stimulate a point known as Stomach 16 (or Ying Chuang or Stop Asthma). Do this twice a day, morning and evening, for the rest of this week.

Stimulating Stomach 16

1 Locate a point just below your third rib, directly above your nipple (see page 36).

2 Press the point on the left-hand side of your chest with your thumb, gradually increasing the pressure, then releasing it when it feels uncomfortable.

3 Build up the pressure again, then slowly release. Repeat a total of five times, then do the same on your right hand side.

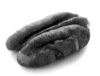

the full-strength program day three

Daily menu

- **Breakfast: Cheesy Mushroom and Egg Risotto (see page 165)**

- **Morning snack: a large apple (Jonathan, Red Delicious or Golden Delicious only)**

- **Lunch: Hummus (see page 166). Toast. Carrot and celery sticks. Low-fat bio yogurt with allowed fruit and nuts**

- **Afternoon snack: handful of Brazil nuts**

- **Dinner: mixed beans, such as chickpeas, soy beans, split peas and kidney beans (but not broad beans), sautéd with onions and garlic, then simmered in Low-Salicylate Vegetable Bouillon (see page 172) with tomatoes, parsnip and carrots. Add saffron and parsley for flavour. Garlic bread. Mango Yogurt Ice Cream (see page 173)**

- **Drinks: 570ml/20fl oz/scant 2^1/$_3$ cups semi-skimmed or skimmed milk. Camomile tea, rosehip tea and mineral water. One glass of grapefruit, pineapple or carrot juice**

- **Supplements: see page 145**

Daily breathing exercise

Today's technique is alternate nostril breathing. It cleanses and purifies the respiratory passages and relaxes your airways. Do this for one minute, twice a day.

Alternate nostril breathing

1 Bring your right hand to your nose, so your right thumb can easily close your right nostril, and your right index finger can easily close your left nostril. You're going to alternately block and release your nostrils as you breathe.

2 Close your right nostril with your right thumb and breathe in through your left nostril. Then, close your left nostril with your right index finger while, at the same time, releasing your thumb from the right nostril and exhaling through it.

3 Inhale through your right nostril, then close your right nostril with your right thumb and exhale through your left nostril.

Acupressure

Stimulate the acupressure points from days one and two, and then, using the steps below, stimulate

Lung 1 (also known as Zhong Fu or Letting Go). Do this for two minutes, twice a day, morning and evening, for the rest of this week.

Stimulating Lung 1

1 Find the points on the top of your chest, under your collar bone (see page 36).

2 Let your head drop forward, then breathe in through your nose and out through your mouth as you press the points on each side with your thumbs.

3 Build up the pressure until it feels uncomfortable, then slowly release.

Brain power

Alternate nostril breathing is thought to bring balance to brain function. Researchers have found that, when the right nostril is closed, electrical activity in the right side of the brain increases, which helps you perform creative, or right-brain tasks. When the left nostril is closed, you perform better in verbal or left-brain skills.

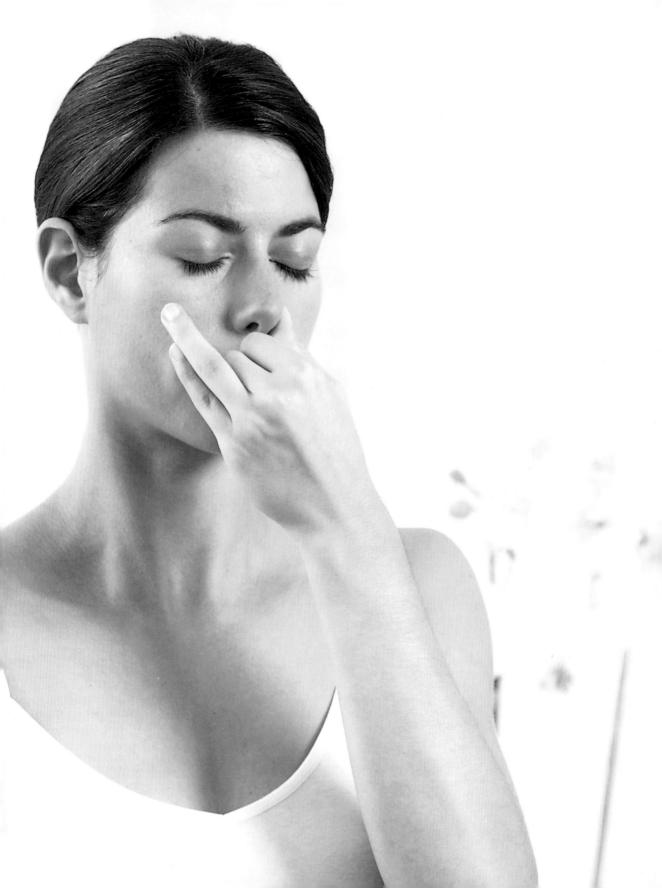

the full-strength program day four

Daily menu

- **Breakfast: grilled tomatoes on toast**

- **Morning snack: a large apple (Jonathan, Red Delicious or Golden Delicious only)**

- **Lunch: Waldorf Salad (chopped walnuts, Red Delicious apple and celery with yogurt). Bowl of lettuce with chopped tomatoes and red onion, drizzled with olive oil and lemon juice and sprinkled with coriander leaves, parsley and chives. Bread. Low-fat bio yogurt with allowed fruit and nuts**

- **Afternoon snack: handful of pecans**

- **Dinner: Grilled Chicken Breasts with Lemon and Herbs (see page 168). Corn on the cob. Braised leeks. Brown rice. Grilled banana topped with chopped walnuts and crème fraîche**

- **Drinks: 570ml/20fl oz/scant 2^1/$_3$ cups semi-skimmed or skimmed milk. Camomile tea, rosehip tea and mineral water. One glass of grapefruit, pineapple or carrot juice**

- **Supplements: see page 145**

Daily breathing exercise

Today, I'd like you to do yesterday's alternate nostril breathing technique followed by bee breath, which has a soothing, calming effect.

Bee breath

1   Take a slow, deep breath through your nose. Exhale through both nostrils and make a soft buzzing in your throat.
2   Do this five times, making the sound louder with each breath.

Acupressure

Stimulate the acupressure points from days one to three and then stimulate Urinary Bladder 13 (also known as Feishu or Lung Transport). Do this for two minutes, twice a day, morning and evening, for the rest of this week.

Stimulating Urinary Bladder 13

1   Find this point between your shoulder blade and spine on each side (see page 36).
2   Press firmly on the point on your left-hand side. Build the pressure to the limit of comfort, then slowly release it. If the point is tricky to access, use a tennis ball – lie on your back with your knees bent. Slip the ball under your shoulder and manipulate it to the right point. Cross your arms over your body and, breathing deeply, let your weight sink onto the ball.
3   Do this five times on the left side, then five times repeat on the right side.

Take echinacea

The herbal remedy echinacea wards off colds and other respiratory infections by increasing the number and activity of white blood cells responsible for fighting both viral and bacterial infections. Research shows that taking echinacea more than halves your chance of catching a cold and, if a cold does develop, symptoms are milder and last around two days less than normal. Take echinacea regularly throughout the winter months (it doesn't contain salicylates). Alternatively, take the herb at a higher dose (see page 27) when you first feel cold symptoms developing.

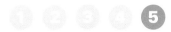

day five

Daily menu

- **Breakfast: muesli with chopped kiwi (follow the recipe on page 132 but omit the almonds, dates and apricots)**

- **Morning snack: a large apple (Jonathan, Red Delicious or Golden Delicious only)**

- **Lunch: Garlic and Sweet Potato Soup (see page 166). Bread roll. Low-fat bio yogurt with allowed fruit and nuts**

- **Afternoon snack: handful of Brazil nuts**

- **Dinner: Cod with Cheesy Couscous (see page 170). Green peas. Cauliflower. Fresh mango**

- **Drinks: 570ml/20fl oz/scant 2$^1/_3$ cups semi-skimmed or skimmed milk. Camomile tea, rosehip tea and mineral water. One glass of grapefruit, pineapple or carrot juice**

- **Supplements: see page 145**

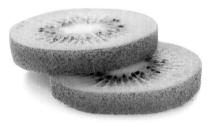

Today's soup contains orange-coloured sweet potatoes, which are one of the richest dietary sources of antioxidant carotenoids. and a good source of vitamins C and E, and fibre. You can also eat them mashed, roasted or baked – just like a normal potato, but without the salicylates.

Daily breathing exercise

Start with alternate nostril breathing from day three and then do the following pranayama: dirgha or three-part breath.

Three-part breath

1 Sit upright but relaxed. Close your eyes and, as you breathe in though your nose and out through your mouth, focus on the expansion and contraction of your belly and ribcage. As you breathe out, let tension fall away so your abdomen drops.

2 Next, breathe in as fully as you can – let your belly swell first, then let your ribcage expand, and finally feel the upper part of your lungs expanding with air to make your collar bones rise.

3 As you breathe out, notice how air first leaves your upper chest, then your midriff and finally your abdomen – contract your abdominal muscles to expel the last bit of air.

Acupressure

Stimulate the acupressure points from days one to four and then stimulate Lung 5 (also known as Foot Marsh). Do this for two minutes, twice a day, morning and evening.

Stimulating Lung 5

1 Find the point on your inner forearm, just below the crease of your elbow on the thumb side of your arm. Feel down the line where there is a visible change in the colour and texture of your skin until you find a point that feels tender. If you can't find an obviously tender point, press 2.5cm (1in) away from your elbow crease.

2 Use your right thumb to press firmly on the point on your left arm. Build up the pressure until it feels uncomfortable, then slowly relax the pressure again. Do this five times on the left side, then repeat on the right side.

the full-strength program day six

Daily menu

- **Breakfast: Mozzarella Eggs (see page 165). Toast**

- **Morning snack: a large apple (Jonathan, Red Delicious or Golden Delicious only)**

- **Lunch: Hummus (see page 166). Toast. Carrot and celery sticks. Low-fat bio yogurt with allowed fruit and nuts**

- **Afternoon snack: handful of pecans**

- **Dinner: Stir-Fried Rice with Vegetables and Peanut Butter Sauce (see page 172). Steamed green cabbage. Kiwi fruit**

- **Drinks: 570ml/20fl oz/scant 2^1/$_3$ cups semi-skimmed or skimmed milk. Camomile tea, rosehip tea and mineral water. One glass of grapefruit, pineapple or carrot juice**

- **Supplements: see page 145**

Daily breathing exercise

Start with the alternate nostril breathing technique to clear your respiratory passages (see day three), and then repeat the three-part breath you did yesterday. As you do the three-part breath, I'd like you to increase the length of both your inhalation and your exhalation. Listen to the sound your breath makes – it should be smooth and harmonious rather than jerky, forced or ragged. Practise the three-part breath for five minutes, or for as long as it feels comfortable.

Acupressure

From now on, I'd like you to repeat the acupressure routine you've learned over the last few days every day for the rest of this program. Alternatively, you may prefer to buy some adhesive magnetic patches and stick one

An underactive thyroid

Some researchers have found that asthma is worse in people with an underactive thyroid gland, and that asthma improves once a thyroid condition is treated. Thyroid problems often go undiagnosed, so it's worth getting a thyroid check if your asthma doesn't respond to dietary and lifestyle changes, and using your medication as prescribed.

over your left and right Stomach 16 acupoints (also known as Stop Asthma); see page 36. These are located on the front of your chest on each side, just below your third rib, and directly above your nipple. Keep the patches in place for five days, then replace every five days for the rest of this program.

Peanut butter

Today's dinner includes peanut butter. If you have a peanut allergy, make a tomato sauce instead using finely chopped beef tomatoes and fresh herbs. You should also avoid eating peanut butter for breakfast on days seven and fourteen.

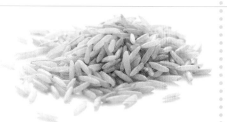

day seven

Daily menu

- **Breakfast: grilled grapefruit. Toast and peanut butter**

- **Morning snack: a large apple (Jonathan, Red Delicious or Golden Delicious only)**

- **Lunch: tuna, green beans and beansprouts drizzled with olive oil and lemon juice and sprinkled with parsley and chives. Bread roll. Low-fat bio yogurt with allowed fruit and nuts**

- **Afternoon snack: handful of Brazil nuts**

- **Dinner: Turkey Stew with Split Peas and Spinach (see page 169). Mashed parsnip and turnips. Plain, uncoloured cheeses with biscuits**

- **Drinks: 570ml/20fl oz/scant 2^1/3 cups semi-skimmed or skimmed milk. Camomile tea, rosehip tea and mineral water. One glass of grapefruit, pineapple or carrot juice**

- **Supplements: see page 145**

Daily breathing exercise

Start with the alternate nostril breathing technique from day three, then do the three-part breath from day five. As you exhale during the three-part breath, make a soft, whispering, "hhhhhhhhh" noise by slightly constricting the back of your throat – as if you're trying to fog up a window. This technique increases the respiratory benefits of the three-part breath by further exercising your diaphragm.

Consulting an acupuncturist

After a week of practising acupressure on yourself, it's now time to visit an acupuncturist for a course of traditional Chinese acupuncture. This can regulate the flow of qi energy in your body, which helps to stabilize your airways and reduce bronchospasm. During a consultation, the practitioner will take your medical history, and examine you – this usually includes looking at your tongue and assessing your pulse (in Traditional Chinese Medicine there are 12 wrist pulses; six on each wrist). Sterile, disposable, slender needles are inserted into your skin at selected acupoints; this should not be uncomfortable. Usually, the acupuncturist will use between six and 12 needles, most commonly selecting points on the hands and feet. The practitioner may stimulate the needles with moxa – a herb – or by applying a small, low-frequency electrical current (electroacupuncture). Some needles are left in position for as little as a few seconds, while others may be left in for 30 minutes or more. To find an accredited acupuncturist, check the resources on page 174.

Fig plants

The decorative indoor weeping fig, *Ficus benjamina*, is a common cause of latex sensitivity. Researchers recommend that people with allergic asthma should not keep *Ficus benjamina* in their homes as it can make asthma worse – even in people who do not have a latex sensitivity.

the full-strength program day eight

Daily menu

- **Breakfast: chopped fresh figs with prosciutto (salt-cured; no spices) and papaya. Bread roll**

- **Morning snack: a large apple (Jonathan, Red Delicious or Golden Delicious only)**

- **Lunch: cold roast turkey. Coleslaw made with shredded cabbage, carrot, spring onion and sweetcorn. Bowl of lettuce, chopped tomato, spring onion and celery, drizzled with olive oil and lemon juice and sprinkled with hazelnuts and coriander leaves. Bread. Low-fat bio yogurt with allowed fruit and nuts**

- **Afternoon snack: handful of pecans**

- **Dinner: Sole Parcels with Oyster Mushrooms (see page 170). Peas. Carrots. Sweet potatoes. Tropical Fruit Salad (see page 173)**

- **Drinks: 570ml/20fl oz/scant 2$^1/_3$ cups semi-skimmed or skimmed milk. Camomile tea, rosehip tea and mineral water. One glass of grapefruit, pineapple or carrot juice**

- **Supplements: see page 145**

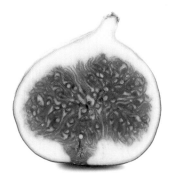

Over the next few days I recommend a number of self-help therapies for you to try – if one of them works particularly well, incorporate it into your life on a daily basis and research other techniques from the same therapy that might also help.

Daily breathing exercise

Do your usual alternate nostril breathing (see day three) followed by the three-part breath (see day five). Today, as you practise the three-part breath, I'd like you to breathe in and out only through your mouth. Make a soft, hissing "sssss" sound as you inhale, and then a whispering "hhhhhhhhh" sound as you exhale. This technique is known as ocean breath because your breathing resembles the sound of waves

washing in and out from the shore. Do this three times.

Aromatherapy

Take an aromatherapy bath that contains a blend of the following anti-spasmodic aromatherapy oils in 15ml carrier oil (see page 25):

- Two drops camomile
- Two drops lavender
- Two drops marjoram

Draw your bath so that it's comfortably warm, then add the oil mixture once the taps are turned off. Keep the lights low, and lie in the fragrant water for 15 minutes, with your eyes closed.

Aerobic exercise
Don't neglect your aerobic exercise routine (see page 68). And remember that if you warm up with several short, 30-second sprints over five or 10 minutes before starting, this seems to protect against exercise-induced asthma for around 40 minutes.

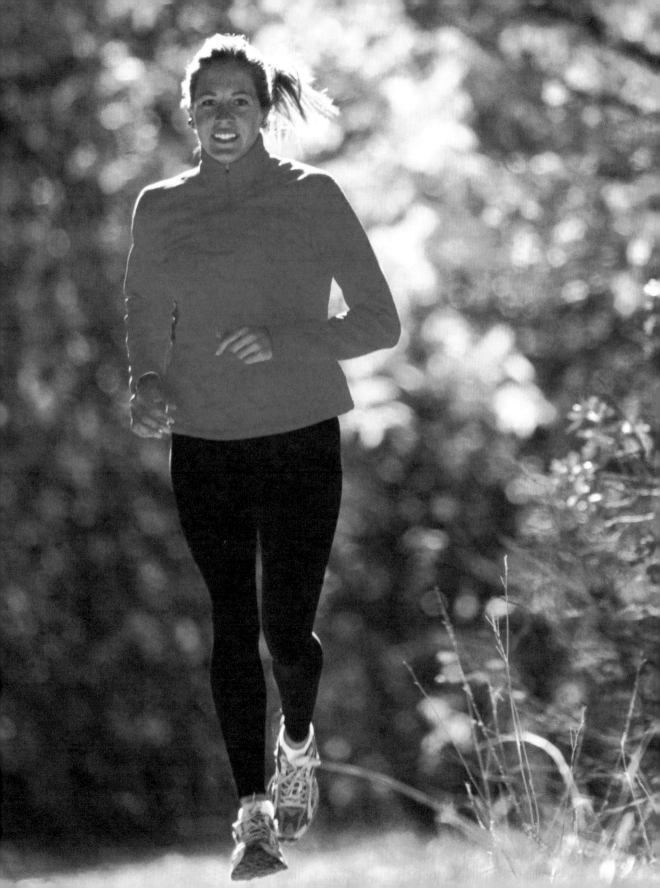

the full-strength program day nine

Daily menu

- **Breakfast: muesli with chopped banana (follow the recipe on page 132 but omit the almonds, dates and apricots)**

- **Morning snack: a large apple (Jonathan, Red Delicious or Golden Delicious only)**

- **Lunch: Mushroom Pâté (see page 167). Toast. Bowl of chopped tomatoes and red onion, drizzled with olive oil and lemon juice, and sprinkled with coriander leaves. Low-fat bio yogurt with allowed fruit and nuts**

- **Afternoon snack: handful of Brazil nuts**

- **Dinner: pasta with green beans, peas, crème fraîche, garlic and parsley sprinkled with Parmesan. Lettuce drizzled with olive oil and lemon juice. Stewed Plums with Pecan Nuts (see page 173)**

- **Drinks: 570ml/20fl oz/scant 2 1/3 cups semi-skimmed or skimmed milk. Camomile tea, rosehip tea and mineral water. One glass of grapefruit, pineapple or carrot juice**

- **Supplements: see page 145**

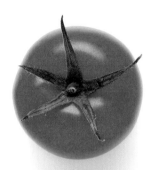

Daily breathing exercise

Do your usual alternate nostril breathing (see day three), followed by today's variation of the three-part breath: instead of making soft, whispering sounds as you did yesterday, make a humming sound that vibrates throughout your body as you breathe out (your mouth can be open or closed). Settle into a sound that resonates well for you – yoga practitioners often use the sacred sound of "om". Making a vibrating sound as you exhale tones and strengthens the diaphragm, and is helpful for people with asthma. Do this for five minutes or for as long as feels comfortable.

Naturopathy

Tonight, I'd like you to try another type of therapeutic bath in which you apply a naturopathic flax seed (linseed) poultice to your chest. Add 250g (9oz) ground flax seeds to 600ml (21fl oz) boiling water and stir continuously. Allow to cool until comfortably warm (caution: poultices retain heat for a long time, so take care not to burn yourself). Put the poultice in a wet tea towel and place this on your chest while you lie in a warm bath for 20 minutes (or, if you prefer, apply the warm poultice directly to your skin and shower afterwards). Alternatively, use an essential oil hot compress as described on page 28.

Ultrasonic remedy

Consider investing in an ultrasonic dust mite controller (check online for products). This is a device that disrupts the feeding and reproductive cycles of the dust mite by emitting a range of ultrasonic sounds (which can't be heard by humans or pets). Clinical trials in Italy have shown that the device reduces population numbers of the dust mite and reduces allergen exposure.

day ten

Daily menu

- **Breakfast: toast. Mushrooms sautéed with garlic, cream and parsley**

- **Morning snack: a large apple (Jonathan, Red Delicious or Golden Delicious only)**

- **Lunch: Beetroot Soup (see opposite). Bread roll. Low-fat bio yogurt with allowed fruit and nuts**

- **Afternoon snack: handful of pecans**

- **Dinner: Lamb Steaks with Parsley and Walnut Crust (see page 169). Steamed spinach (frozen, not fresh). Sweet potatoes. Mango Yogurt Ice Cream (see page 173)**

- **Drinks: 570ml/20fl oz/scant 2^1/₃ cups semi-skimmed or skimmed milk. Camomile tea, rosehip tea and mineral water. One glass of grapefruit, pineapple or carrot juice**

- **Supplements: see page 145**

Today's lunch is beetroot soup, which you can make by cooking beetroot, carrots, onion, celery – or any other vegetable on your allowed list – in Low-Salicylate Vegetable Bouillon (see page 172). Cook the vegetables until they are soft, then purée with the cooking water and flavour with lemon juice and bio yogurt. The purple-red pigments in beetroot include powerful antioxidants that are traditionally used to cleanse the blood and protect against respiratory infections. You can also juice beetroot together with carrots for an antioxidant-rich morning drink.

Daily breathing exercise

After you've practised alternate nostril breathing (see day three), do today's variation of the three-part breath: breathe in through your nose and out through your mouth, making your breath flow seamlessly. When you feel ready, pause and hold your breath for a few seconds after you have inhaled fully. Take a similar pause after you have exhaled fully. Keep doing this for five minutes, or as long as feels comfortable.

Homeopathy

Although it's best to consult a homeopath for individual advice, there are some remedies known as allersodes that are designed to reduce your reaction against common environmental allergens. They contain homeopathic preparations of animal danders, pollens, biting insect venoms, household dust mites or moulds. If you have a known allergy to one of these groups of allergens, buy the appropriate allersode from a homeopathic pharmacy and take 10 drops three times a day to help desensitize yourself. Alternatively, if you consulted a homeopath at the end of the gentle program, continue taking the remedies they prescribed for you.

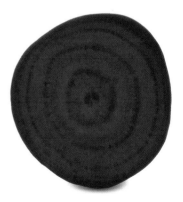

the full-strength program day eleven

Daily menu

- **Breakfast: African la Bouillie (see page 164)**

- **Morning snack: a large apple (Jonathan, Red Delicious or Golden Delicious only)**

- **Lunch: Hummus (see page 166). Toast. Carrot and celery sticks. Low-fat bio yogurt with allowed fruit and nuts**

- **Afternoon snack: handful of Brazil nuts**

- **Dinner: Steamed Monkfish Parcels with Parsley Vinaigrette (see page 170). Braised beetroot. Carrots. Spring greens. Banana and Walnut Bread (see page 173)**

- **Drinks: 570ml/20fl oz/scant 2^1/$_3$ cups semi-skimmed or skimmed milk. Camomile tea, rosehip tea and mineral water. One glass of grapefruit, pineapple or carrot juice**

- **Supplements: see page 145**

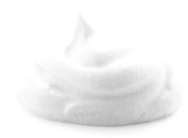

Daily breathing exercise

Today, I'd like to introduce you to the first stage of an advanced breathing technique, called viloma pranayama (meaning "against the natural order"). It involves interrupted breathing. The purpose of stage one is simply to familiarize you with the breathing rhythm – the more therapeutic second stage of the exercise will come tomorrow. Do stage one immediately after today's alternate nostril breathing exercise.

Viloma pranayama, stage 1

1 Lie on your back on a firm surface with your arms relaxed by your sides. Take a few normal breaths then, when you feel ready, inhale for two or three seconds then pause and hold your breath for two or three seconds.

2 Continue to inhale for another two or three seconds and then pause again.

3 Repeat step two until your lungs are full – usually after four to five pauses.

4 Now breathe out slowly and steadily until your lungs feel empty. Breathe normally before repeating the whole exercise once more.

Herbalism

Today I suggest you add a herbal medicine to your supplement regime. The remedy I've selected is a traditional Asian herb known as Chinese basil or wild coleus (*Perilla frutescens*) that has a powerful anti-allergy action. Studies in Japan and Finland show that at least 80 percent of those using it find it helpful against symptoms of perennial allergy, such as recurrent sneezing, watery or itchy nose and eyes, and facial itching. See page 26 for dosage instructions. If your asthma has not improved as much as you would like on the full-strength program, you could also try taking frankincense (*Boswellia serrata*). See page 25 for dosage instructions.

day twelve

Daily menu

- Breakfast: muesli with chopped Williams pear (follow the recipe on page 132 but omit the almonds, dates and apricots)

- Morning snack: a large apple (Jonathan, Red Delicious or Golden Delicious only)

- Lunch: Mussel and Leek Soup (see page 167). Bread roll. Low-fat bio yogurt with allowed fruit and nuts

- Afternoon snack: handful of pecans

- Dinner: stir-fried rice with beansprouts, bamboo shoots (canned), carrots, sweetcorn and mushrooms (flavour with garlic, soy sauce and coriander leaves). Rhubarb and Banana Fool (see page 173)

- Drinks: 570ml/20fl oz/scant $2^1/3$ cups semi-skimmed or skimmed milk. Camomile tea, rosehip tea and mineral water. One glass of grapefruit, pineapple or carrot juice

- Supplements: see page 145

Daily breathing exercise

Below I describe the second part of viloma pranayama. Whereas stage 1 (see day eleven) involved interrupted inhalations, stage 2 involves interrupted exhalations and is more therapeutic. It has a beneficial effect on both your circulation and your respiratory system. Do alternate nostril breathing first.

Viloma pranayama, stage 2

1 Lie on your back on a firm surface with your arms relaxed by your sides. When you feel ready, breathe out completely, then inhale smoothly until your lungs feel full.

2 Breathe out slowly for two or three seconds and pause, holding your breath for two or three seconds. Breathe out for a further two or three seconds before pausing again.

3 Keep doing these exhalations and pauses until your lungs feel empty – this usually takes four or five pauses. Breathe in and out normally a few times, then repeat the interrupted exhalations. Do this five times in total.

Meditation

Today spend 15 minutes focusing your mind on a mandala to help you relax – a mandala is a diagram whose name derives from the Sanskrit word for circle. Choose one that appeals to you from www.mandalaproject.org. To contemplate your mandala sit quietly and comfortably and clear your mind of thought. Let your gaze absorb the colours, shapes and textures of your mandala.

Use a salt pipe

Inhaling through a salt pipe for a few minutes each day allows you to practise speleotherapy (see page 62) in your own home. Salt pipes are made from porcelain and contain salt crystals from the Transylvanian Praid salt mine. As you breathe in through the pipe, air is moisturized and also picks up micron-sized salt particles that cleanse and stabilize your respiratory passages, as well as thinning the mucus in your airways so it becomes easier to expel.

the full-strength program
day thirteen

Daily menu

- **Breakfast: Spinach and Leek Frittata with Tomato Salad (see page 165)**

- **Morning snack: a large apple (Jonathan, Red Delicious or Golden Delicious only)**

- **Lunch: Split Pea Dip (see page 166). Toast. Bowl of lettuce leaves, chopped tomatoes and red onion drizzled with olive oil and lemon juice. Low-fat bio yogurt with allowed fruit and nuts**

- **Afternoon snack: handful of Brazil nuts**

- **Dinner: Normandy Chicken with Creamed Apples and Cider (see page 168). Cauliflower. Carrots. Green beans. Fresh papaya**

- **Drinks: 570ml/20fl oz/scant 2$\frac{1}{3}$ cups semi-skimmed or skimmed milk. Camomile tea, rosehip tea and mineral water. One glass of grapefruit, pineapple or carrot juice**

- **Supplements: see page 145**

Daily breathing exercise

This is an advanced breathing technique called kapalabhati (breath of fire), which is said to have a purifying effect on the lungs. It involves a passive inhalation, followed by an active, forced exhalation. Practise it after alternate nostril breathing.

Breath of fire

1 Inhale through your nose, then force the air out as quickly as you can, as if blowing out a candle through your nose. Put your hand on your abdomen so you can feel your muscles actively pumping out air.
2 Repeat this breath 10 times, in a quick, steady rhythm. Build up to doing more once you become experienced.

Visualization

Today I'd like you to find a quiet and comfortable place in which to lie down and do the following visualization.

Oxygen visualization

1 Lie on your back on an exercise mat with your arms resting a little way from your body,

Cat allergens

A large European study suggests that increasing exposure to cat allergens can worsen bronchoconstriction triggered by other allergens, even in adults whose blood tests show they are not allergic to cats. This suggests that all allergic individuals show signs of asthma in response to cat allergen – for this reason you may find it helpful to limit your exposure to cats.

palms facing up. Let your feet fall to the sides. Breathe in slowly through your nose, and out through your mouth.
2 As you inhale, visualize oxygen as a bright, white, calming light entering your body and flowing through your lungs, and then out to the rest of your body, before exiting smoothly through your mouth.
3 Stay focused on the light as it enters and leaves your body. Do this for 15 minutes, and notice how calm and relaxed your feel afterwards.

day fourteen

Daily menu

- **Breakfast: grilled grapefruit. Toast and peanut butter**

- **Morning snack: a large apple (Jonathan, Red Delicious or Golden Delicious only)**

- **Lunch: bowl of chopped celery and red onion, beans and grated carrot drizzled with olive oil and lemon juice and sprinkled with garlic and coriander leaves. Coleslaw (see menu, page 154). Bread roll. Low-fat bio yogurt with allowed fruit and nuts**

- **Afternoon snack: handful of pecans**

- **Dinner: tagliatelle with bacon, peas, crème fraîche, garlic and parsley sprinkled with Parmesan. Bowl of lettuce, chopped tomatoes and red onions drizzled with olive oil and lemon juice. Tropical Fruit Salad (see page 173)**

- **Drinks: 570ml/20fl oz/scant 2^1/$_3$ cups semi-skimmed or skimmed milk. Camomile tea, rosehip tea and mineral water. One glass of grapefruit, pineapple or carrot juice**

- **Supplements: see page 145**

Try eating little and often throughout the day – so rather than eating your bread roll and yogurt with your salad at lunch, try spreading the meal out over two or three hours. Eating a whole meal in one sitting can contribute to shortness of breath because a full stomach puts pressure on the diaphragm, making it difficult to breathe in fully.

Daily breathing exercise

Today's exercise helps you relax and can significantly improve your asthma control. Do it after alternate nostril breathing when you're in bed at the beginning and end of the day.

The complete breath

1 Lie on your back with your arms relaxed by your sides. Close your eyes and breathe slowly in and out through your nose. Spend twice as long breathing out as you do breathing in.

2 Raise both arms above your head as you breathe in as if you are reaching up into the sky. Visualize your lungs filling with oxygen.

3 As you slowly breathe out, lower your arms back down to your sides and relax. Repeat five times.

Consulting a nutritional therapist

If you have followed all three programs in this book, you will have increased your intake of anti-inflammatory antioxidants and omega-3 fatty acids (the gentle program), eliminated dietary sulfites (the moderate program) and reduced your intake of salicylates (the full-strength program). If, despite these approaches, your asthma is not as controlled as you want it to be, you may have an idiosyncratic food intolerance. Try consulting a naturopath or nutritional therapist who specializes in food intolerances; and have a blood test that incubates your live white blood cells with food extracts (see pages 44–45). Another blood test that may prove helpful is one that looks for raised levels of anti-food IgG antibodies (see page 44). A nutritional therapist can also advise you about the type of elimination diet that may now be useful.

continuing the full-strength program

Now that you've followed the full-strength program for a month, you need to assess whether or not reducing your exposure to dietary salicylates has improved your asthma symptoms. If you haven't noticed a significant benefit, try following either the gentle or the moderate program. Or, if you've already tried the gentle and moderate programs, it's likely that a component of your diet (apart from an imbalance between omega-6s and omega-3s, or exposure to dietary sulfites or salicylates) is affecting your asthma control. Please see my advice on page 161 about consulting a nutritional therapist.

If you *have* noticed a significant improvement in your asthma over the last month, then it's likely that you're sensitive to dietary salicylates and you should aim to minimize your exposure to foods containing high amounts of these in the future. Remember to also exclude any other foods you have identified as triggering your asthma symptoms. Now you have an understanding of the diet and lifestyle changes you need to make, you can start to plan your own diet while taking into account your likes and dislikes.

Your long-term diet

Continue to eat healthily – lots of fresh fruit and vegetables, selected nuts and oily fish – while minimizing your exposure to the dietary salicylates that are naturally present in some foods. Because you are sensitive to these aspirin-like substances, you need to be fully aware of the foods that contain them. You also need to be aware of the foods that contain the food colouring tartrazine, and exclude these from your diet

(tartrazine and salicylate sensitivities tend to be linked). If you're in any doubt about the foods you should avoid or eat in moderation, go back and re-read the charts on pages 47 and 49. Get into the habit of always checking ingredients lists when buying ready-made foods. Take care to eat only certain types of apple and, in particular, avoid "banned" herbs and spices, many of which contain exceptionally high amounts of salicylates. You should also check with a pharmacist or doctor before taking any over-the-counter or prescribed medicines to ensure they are salicylate-free. If you eat a food containing salicylates, you risk developing symptoms such as those described on page 48, as well as experiencing an asthma attack.

Fortunately, there are plenty of foods that you're able to eat in your daily diet – use the shopping list on page 144 as a basic list and add your own food choices to it. Concentrate on eating at least four or five servings of salad stuff and vegetables (not including potatoes) and two or three servings of fruit a day as snacks. Vary the fruit and vegetables in your diet; aim for a rainbow of colours on your plate wherever possible.

Research recipes that contain salicylate-free foods, especially fish-based and vegetarian recipes. You will find some recipe suggestions on my website (www.naturalhealthguru.co.uk) and you can post your own favourites there, too, for other followers of the full-strength program to try.

If the full-strength program diet works for you, and your asthma symptoms are well controlled, aim to follow its principles for the rest of your life.

Your long-term supplement regime

Continue taking the recommended supplements for the full-strength program (see page 145) long term. Research supports their use at this high level for significant beneficial effects on lung function and asthma symptoms. If you've taken only the supplements in the "desirable" list, you may like to add in one or more of the supplements in the "optional" list for extra benefit. Alternatively, if your asthma symptoms are well controlled, you may wish to reduce the dose of your supplements back down to the levels suggested in the moderate program. If, after a month, your symptoms are still well controlled, you can step down your supplement doses to those recommended in the gentle program. This stepping down of your supplements is similar in principle to the stepping down of the asthma treatments that your doctor or practice nurse has devised for you in your personal asthma management plan (see pages 20–21).

Your exercise routine

The daily pranayama breath control exercises in the full-strength program should have improved your lung function. Continue to do these exercises or, if you prefer, do those based on the Buteyko method, which I have included in the moderate program, or the basic breath control techniques I suggested in the gentle program. You should also continue to do at least 30 minutes of brisk aerobic exercise on most days, for example, walking, swimming or cycling. Build up to exercising for longer periods as and when you feel ready. Increasing your level of physical exercise is especially important to maintain heart and lung health, and to help you gain and maintain a long-term healthy weight. Do your exercise in two daily sessions of 15 minutes or three daily sessions of 10 minutes if you find this easier – multiple short sessions are just as good for your fitness levels as one longer session. If

Testing for food intolerances

If you consult a complementary therapist about diagnosing food intolerances, a word of caution: although some people have found them useful, there is little evidence to support the use of VEGA electrodermal testing, applied kinesiology, or hair mineral analysis, and I don't personally recommend them. The blood tests I mention on page 161 have more evidence to support their efficacy.

exercise triggers your asthma, follow the tips I've given on pages 68–69 to help overcome this problem.

Your therapy program

The full-strength program has shown you how to use acupressure to benefit your breathing, and introduced you to several other complementary therapies, including aromatherapy, naturopathy, herbal medicine, meditation and visualization. Continue to use the therapies that you have found most beneficial, and continue to consult an acupuncturist if you found the treatment useful. You may also want to explore some of the other therapies I've included in Part Two, such as the Alexander Technique, Rolfing and Hellerwork.

Monitoring your asthma

Continue to record your peak flow measurements on a chart (see page 77). This will give you warning if your asthma control is starting to deteriorate. Ideally, your peak flow readings should stay within 20 percent of your personal best reading (see pages 16–17). If your readings fall below 20 percent of your personal best, seek advice from your doctor or asthma nurse. Also, check to see if you have inadvertently included a source of salicylates or tartrazine in your diet.

breakfast recipes

prosciutto with mango and passion fruit relish

. . . .

serves 4

2 mangoes, peeled, stoned and flesh
   chopped
1 small passion fruit
1 tbsp extra virgin olive oil
Juice of 1 lemon
8 slices prosciutto di Parma*
1 tbsp chopped parsley, to serve

1 In a food processor, purée
    two thirds of the mango
    flesh together with the
    passion fruit pulp.

2 While the food processor is still
    running, slowly add the oil and
    lemon juice.
3 Fold the remaining mango
    into the fruit purée.
4 Put the prosciutto and relish on
    4 plates and sprinkle with the
    parsley, then serve.

* Use true prosciutto di Parma,
which is air-cured using only salt
– no nitrates or spices.

african la bouillie

. . . .

serves 4

200g/7oz/1 cup rice
55g/2oz/scant ¼ cup peanut butter
25g/1oz/scant ¼ cup plain flour
Juice and zest of 1 unwaxed lemon
A little milk or sugar, to serve (optional)

1 Bring the rice and 750ml/26fl
    oz/3 cups water to the boil.
2 Blend the peanut butter and
    flour with 250ml/9fl oz/1 cup
    water to make a paste.
3 Add the peanut-butter mixture
    to the cooking rice. Bring back
    to the boil, then simmer gently,
    uncovered (follow packet
    instructions for cooking time).
4 When the rice is nearly cooked,
    remove it from the heat, stir
    in the lemon juice and zest
    and cover.
5 Stir in some milk and/or sugar,
    according to preference, and
    serve warm.

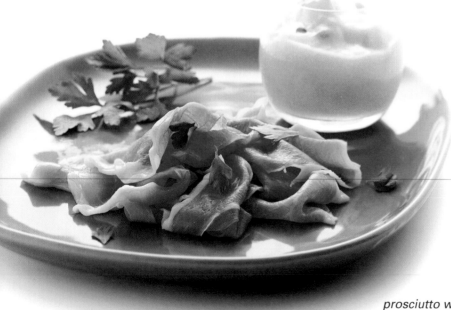

prosciutto with mango and passion fruit relish

cheesy mushroom and egg risotto

serves 4

1 small onion, chopped
1 celery stick, chopped
4 mushrooms, sliced
15g/½oz butter
4 large eggs, beaten
125ml/4fl oz/½ cup semi-skimmed milk
400g/14oz/2 cups cooked brown rice
115g/4oz/1 cup grated plain uncoloured
   Cheddar cheese
1 handful parsley, chopped

1 Sauté the onion, celery and mushrooms in the butter for 2 minutes.
2 Whisk together the eggs and milk and pour over the vegetables. Continue stirring for 2 minutes.
3 Add the rice and cheese and heat through for a further 2 minutes, stirring gently to separate the grains. Serve sprinkled with the parsley.

spinach and leek frittata with tomato salad

serves 4

Juice of ½ lemon
3 tbsp olive oil
1 spring onion, chopped
4 tomatoes, skinned, deseeded
   and chopped
2 baby leeks, chopped
115g/4oz frozen spinach, chopped
6 large eggs
60ml/2fl oz/¼ cup semi-skimmed milk
115g/4oz plain feta cheese, crumbled
1 handful parsley, chopped

1 Whisk together the lemon juice and half the olive oil. Add the spring onion and tomatoes.
2 Cook the leeks in boiling water for 1 minute. Add the spinach and cook for a further 1 minute. Drain, rinse and pat dry.
3 Whisk together the eggs and milk and mix with the leeks, spinach and feta cheese.
4 Preheat the grill to high. Heat the remaining oil in an oven-proof pan and add the egg mixture. Fry for 5 minutes, then grill until the top is golden.
5 Sprinkle with the parsley and serve with the tomato salad.

mozzarella eggs

serves 4

15g/½oz butter
4 large eggs
1 handful chives, chopped
4 slices plain mozzarella cheese

1 Melt the butter in a frying pan. When hot, slide the eggs into the pan, one at a time.
2 Cook for 2 minutes, or until the whites are set, then sprinkle with some of the chives. Put a slice of mozzarella on each egg, then sprinkle with the remaining chives.
3 Add 1½ teaspoons water to the pan, remove from the heat, cover and leave to stand 5 minutes before serving.

lunch recipes

hummus

serves 4

150g/5½oz/²⁄₃ cup dried chickpeas, soaked overnight, then rinsed and drained
4 tbsp extra virgin olive oil
Juice and zest of 2 unwaxed lemons
3 garlic cloves, crushed
115g/4oz light tahini (sesame) paste*
Rock salt
1 tbsp chopped parsley, to serve

1 Simmer the chickpeas in water for 1½ hours, or until soft. Drain, saving the cooking liquid.
2 Put 80ml/2½fl oz/¹⁄₃ cup of the cooking liquid in a food processor with the olive oil, lemon juice, zest and garlic. Blend, gradually adding the chickpeas and tahini paste. If the food processor clogs, add more liquid until the mixture forms a grainy, creamy purée. Season with salt.
3 Add more olive oil or tahini paste to vary the flavour as desired.

* Make sure the tahini contains only sesame seeds and no banned ingredients.

split pea dip

serves 4

225g/8oz/1 cup yellow split peas
1 onion, chopped
3 garlic cloves, crushed
1.2l/44fl oz/5 cups water
4 tbsp extra virgin olive oil
Juice and zest of 1 unwaxed lemon
Wholemeal pitta bread, to serve

1 Place the split peas, onion and garlic in a large pan with 1.2l/44fl oz/5 cups water. Bring to a boil, skim off any foam, cover and simmer gently for 1 hour until the peas absorb the water.
2 Beat the olive oil into the peas to form a purée.
3 Add the lemon juice and zest and serve with pitta bread.

garlic and sweet potato soup

serves 4

1 whole bulb of garlic, halved horizontally
2 onions, finely chopped
2 celery sticks, finely chopped
2 carrots, finely chopped
15g/½oz butter
4 orange-fleshed sweet potatoes, peeled and chopped
600ml/1pt/2¹⁄₃ cups Low-Salicylate Vegetable Bouillon (see page 172) or chicken stock (made with bones only)
300ml/10½fl oz/1¹⁄₄ cups skimmed or semi-skimmed milk
1 handful coriander or parsley leaves, chopped

1 Preheat the oven to 200°C/400°F/Gas 6. Roast the garlic for 30 minutes.
2 Sauté the onions, celery and carrots in the butter until soft. Add the sweet potatoes. Cook for 2 minutes. Add the stock and roasted garlic and bring to the boil. Simmer for 30 minutes.
3 Remove the garlic bulbs and scoop out the soft cloves. Purée the soup and garlic cloves in a blender.
4 Reheat and stir in the milk to achieve your preferred consistency. Sprinkle with the coriander or parsley and serve.

mussel and leek soup

. . . .

serves 4

700g/1lb 9oz baby leeks, chopped
15g/½oz butter
1l/35fl oz/4 cups Low-Salicylate
  Vegetable Bouillon (see page 172)
Juice and zest of 1 unwaxed lemon
900g/2lb live mussels, scrubbed and
  debearded (discard any that aren't
  firmly closed)
2 tbsp double cream
1 handful parsley, chopped
1 handful chives, chopped

1 Sauté the leeks in the butter
   until tender.
2 Add the bouillon and lemon
   juice and zest and bring to
   the boil.
3 Add the mussels and simmer
   gently for 5–7 minutes until all
   the mussels open. Shake the
   pan occasionally.
4 Discard any mussels that
   don't open. Add the cream,
   sprinkle the parsley and
   chives on top and serve.

mushroom pâté

. . . .

serves 4

175g/6oz brown mushrooms, finely
  chopped
1 celery stick, finely chopped
1 handful chives, chopped
1 garlic clove, crushed
1 tbsp olive oil
Juice of ½ lemon
100g/3½oz soft cheese
1 anchovy
1 tbsp chopped parsley or chives
Toast, to serve

1 Sauté the mushrooms, celery,
   chives and garlic in the olive oil
   for 10 minutes, or until most of
   the liquid has evaporated.
2 Stir in the lemon juice.
3 Whiz together with the
   remaining ingredients in a
   food processor to make a
   smooth pâté.
4 Serve on toast, sprinkled with
   the parsley or chives.

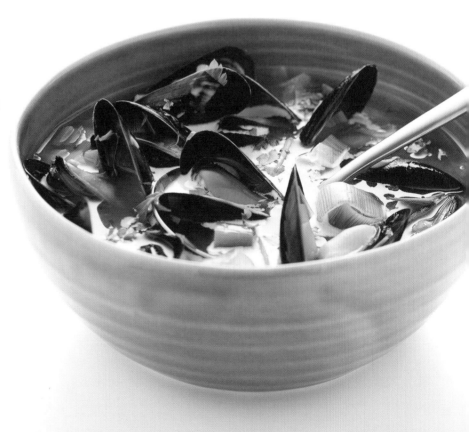

mussel and leek soup

dinner recipes

normandy chicken with creamed apples and cider

. . . .

serves 4

15g/½oz butter
1 tbsp olive oil
1 chicken
3 Golden Delicious apples, peeled,
    cored and sliced
12 shallots, peeled
150ml/5fl oz/scant ⅔ cup Low-Salicylate
    Vegetable Bouillon (see page 172) or
    chicken stock (made with bones only)
300ml/10½fl oz/1¼ cups dry cider
1 handful parsley, chopped
150ml/5fl oz/⅔ cup crème fraîche

1 Preheat the oven to
   180°C/350°F/Gas 4. Heat the
   butter and oil in a flame-proof
   dish and brown the chicken on
   all sides. Remove the chicken,
   fry the apples and shallots
   until coloured, then remove
   and reserve.
2 Return the chicken to the
   casserole and add the bouillon,
   cider and parsley.
3 Bring to the boil, cover, then
   bake for 45 minutes. Add the
   apples and shallots to the
   casserole and cook for a further
   35 minutes, or until the chicken
   is cooked.
4 Remove the chicken and keep
   warm. Stir the crème fraîche

into the cooking liquid and
boil until reduced in volume
by about one third, then serve
with the chicken.

grilled chicken breasts with lemon and herbs

. . . .

serves 4

Juice and zest of 2 unwaxed lemons
1 handful parsley, chopped
1 handful chives, chopped
3 tbsp olive oil
1 garlic clove, crushed
4 chicken breasts

1 Mix together the lemon juice
   and zest, herbs, oil and garlic.
2 Pour the marinade over the
   chicken breasts and leave in
   the fridge for at least 1 hour,
   and preferably overnight.
3 Barbecue or grill the chicken for
   8–10 minutes on each side until
   cooked through and the juices
   run clear, then serve.

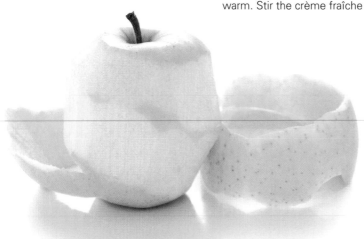

turkey stew with split peas and spinach

serves 4

85g/3oz/⅓ cup green split peas, soaked
    overnight, then rinsed and drained
2 onions, chopped
1 celery stick, chopped
15g/½oz butter
30g/1oz/scant ¼ cup pearl barley
1l/35fl oz/4 cups Low-Salicylate
    Vegetable Bouillon (see page 172) or
    turkey stock (made with bones only)
2 sweet potatoes or parsnips, chopped
4 carrots, chopped
200g/7oz cooked turkey, diced
150g/5½oz frozen spinach, chopped
1 handful coriander leaves, chopped

1 Cover the split peas with water
   and bring to the boil. Simmer
   for 10 minutes, then drain and
   discard the liquid.
2 Sauté the onions and celery
   in the butter until soft.
3 Add the split peas, pearl barley
   and bouillon. Bring to the boil
   and simmer for 40 minutes.
4 Add the sweet potato and
   carrots and simmer for
   15 minutes until tender.
5 Add the turkey and spinach
   and bring back to the boil.
   Sprinkle with the coriander
   and serve.

lamb steaks with parsley and walnut crust

serves 4

55g/2oz/½ cup walnuts, chopped
55g/2oz/⅔ cup fresh white breadcrumbs
1 handful parsley, chopped
2 garlic cloves, crushed
1 tbsp olive oil, plus extra for brushing
4 lamb leg steaks

1 Preheat the oven to
   190°C/375°F/Gas 5. Blend the
   walnuts, breadcrumbs, parsley,
   garlic and olive oil in a food
   processor for 30 seconds.
2 Brush the lamb steaks all over
   with the olive oil and quickly
   sauté over a high heat until
   brown.
3 Transfer the lamb steaks to
   a baking tray and sprinkle
   each one with a quarter of
   the walnut mixture, packing it
   down to make a crust. Bake for
   15–18 minutes until the topping
   is crisp and golden, then serve.

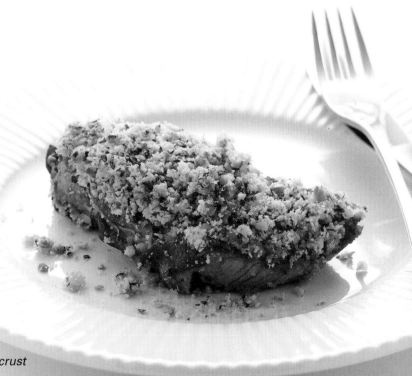

lamb steaks with parsley and walnut crust

cod with cheesy couscous

serves 4

55g/2oz/¹/₃ cup couscous
85g/3oz Parmesan, grated
1 tbsp olive oil
4 cod fillets

1. Soak the couscous in 80ml/
   2½fl oz/²/₃ cup boiling water for
   15 minutes, then stir in the
   Parmesan cheese.
2. Lightly brush a grill pan with
   the olive oil. Put the fish in
   the pan and sprinkle couscous on top.
3. Grill the fish for 10–14 minutes,
   or until cooked, then serve.

steamed monkfish parcels with parsley vinaigrette

serves 4

8 large green cabbage leaves
2 tbsp white wine
Juice and zest of 1 unwaxed lemon
2 shallots, finely chopped
4 monkfish fillets

For the vinaigrette:
1 handful parsley and chives, chopped
1 tbsp malt vinegar
4 tbsp extra virgin olive oil

1. Blanch the cabbage leaves in
   boiling water for 30 seconds.
   Drain and rinse in cold water,
   then pat dry. Remove any
   tough stalks.
2. Put the wine, lemon juice and
   zest, and shallots in a small
   pan. Simmer gently until tender
   and most of the liquid has
   evaporated.
3. Put 2 cabbage leaves on a
   chopping board so they overlap.
   Place a quarter of the shallot
   mixture on the leaves and place
   the monkfish fillet on top. Wrap
   the cabbage leaves around the
   fish to make a parcel. Repeat to
   make 4 parcels.
4. Place the parcels on a steamer
   above simmering water and
   cover. Steam for 15 minutes
   until the fish is cooked.
5. Meanwhile, whisk together the
   vinaigrette ingredients. Drizzle
   a spoonful of vinaigrette over
   each parcel and serve.

sole parcels with oyster mushrooms

serves 4

125g/4½oz oyster mushrooms, finely
   sliced
1 tbsp olive oil
4 spring onions, chopped
Juice and zest of 1 unwaxed lime
4 double fillets lemon sole, skinned
1 handful parsley, chopped

1. Preheat the oven to
   200°C/400°F/Gas 6. Cut out
   4 greaseproof paper circles,
   each 30cm/12in in diameter.
   Fold them in half.
2. Sauté the mushrooms in the
   olive oil for 3 minutes, then add
   the spring onions and cook for
   another 1 minute. Stir in the
   lime zest.
3. Put a fish fillet on each circle
   of greaseproof paper. Put
   a quarter of the mushroom
   mixture along the side of each
   fillet. Sprinkle with the lime
   juice and parsley.
4. Fold the fillet over on top of
   the filling and fold the edges
   of the paper over, pinching
   and tucking to form a sealed
   parcel. Bake in the oven for
   15 minutes, then serve.

right: steamed monkfish parcels with parsley vinaigrette

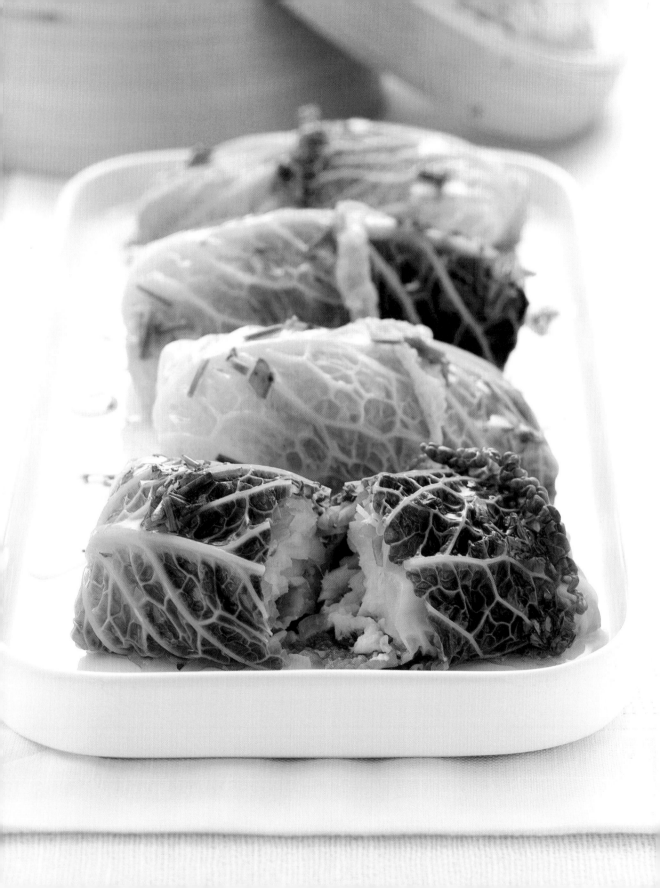

linguini with a saffron prov sauce

serves 4

450g/1lb large prawns, shelled and
    cooked (reserve the shells)
1 unwaxed lemon, sliced
1 onion, chopped
150ml/5fl oz/scant $^2/_3$ cup semi-skimmed
    milk
1 large pinch saffron
450g/1lb fresh, plain linguini pasta or
    350g/12oz dried pasta
1 tbsp olive oil
1 tbsp wholemeal flour
1 handful coriander leaves, chopped

1 To make the stock, put the
    prawn shells, lemon, onion and
    300ml/10½fl oz/1¼ cups water
    in a pan. Bring to the boil and
    simmer for 15 minutes. Strain
    and reserve the liquid.
2 Put the milk and saffron in a
    small pan and bring almost
    to the boil, stirring regularly.
    Remove from the heat and
    leave to infuse for 15 minutes.
3 Cook the pasta according to the
    packet instructions.
4 Heat the oil, add the flour and
    cook for 1 minute, stirring. Add
    the milk and broth, bring to a
    boil and simmer for 1 minute,
    stirring.
5 Add the prawns and coriander
    and cook for a further minute.
    Mix in the pasta and serve.

stir-fried rice with vegetables and peanut butter sauce

serves 4

125g/4½oz/$^2/_3$ cup basmati rice
2 garlic cloves, crushed
1 large carrot, cut into thin strips
70g/2½oz/1 cup shredded red cabbage
200g/7oz canned bamboo shoots,
    drained
12 baby sweetcorn
1 handful mangetout
4 spring onions, chopped
1 tbsp olive oil
2 tbsp light soy sauce
2 tbsp sweet cider
125g/4½oz beansprouts
1 tbsp chopped coriander leaves

For the peanut butter sauce:
2 shallots, finely chopped
2 garlic cloves, crushed
1 tsp olive oil
140g/5oz/scant $^2/_3$ cup smooth peanut
    butter
1 handful coriander, chopped

1 To make the peanut butter
    sauce, sauté the shallots and
    garlic in the oil until soft. Stir
    in the peanut butter and 1½
    cups water. Simmer gently
    for 5 minutes. Blend with the
    coriander in a food processor.
2 Cook the rice according to
    packet instructions, then drain.
3 Sauté the garlic, carrot, red
    cabbage, bamboo shoots, baby
    sweetcorn, mangetout and

spring onions in the olive oil
for 2 minutes.
4 Add the rice, soy sauce and
    cider and stir-fry for a further
    3 minutes.
5 Add the beansprouts and heat
    through. Sprinkle the coriander
    on top and serve with the
    peanut sauce.

low-salicylate vegetable bouillon

makes 3l/105fl oz/12 cups

Make a large batch of this bouillon
and freeze it in small bags.

6 carrots, peeled and roughly chopped
3 onions, peeled and roughly chopped
3 leeks, roughly chopped
3 celery sticks, roughly chopped
6 parsley sprigs, including stems
1 bunch chives, chopped
1 lettuce, roughly chopped

1 Put all the ingredients and
    3.5l/122fl oz/14 cups water in a
    large stockpot, cover and bring
    to the boil. Skim off any scum.
    Simmer gently for 1 hour.
2 Leave to cool slightly before
    straining through a sieve.
    To make a cloudy bouillon
    push some of the ingredients
    through the sieve.

dessert recipes

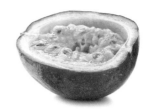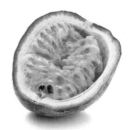

banana and walnut bread

serves 4

115g/4oz butter
55g/2oz/¼ cup sugar
2 large eggs, beaten
175g/6oz/1½ cups self-raising flour, sieved
3 ripe bananas, peeled and mashed
55g/2oz/½ cup walnuts, chopped
A little milk, if needed
Crème fraîche, to serve (optional)

1   Preheat the oven to 180°C/350°F/Gas 4. Beat the butter and sugar together until fluffy. Add the eggs slowly, adding a little flour if the mix curdles. Beat well.
2   Add half the bananas to the mixture. Stir in half the flour, then add the remaining bananas and the walnuts. Fold in the remaining flour. Add a little milk if needed – the mixture should be stiff but able to fall off a spoon.
3   Put the mixture in a non-stick loaf tin and bake for 45 minutes, or until a skewer inserted into the centre comes out clean. Leave to cool. Serve with or without crème fraîche.

stewed plums with pecan nuts

serves 4

700g/25oz/1lb 9oz plums, stoned and sliced
55g/2oz/⅓ cup brown sugar
1 handful pecan nuts, chopped
100g/3½oz/½ cup crème fraîche

1   Put the plums and sugar in a pan and cook over a low heat for 10 minutes.
2   Sprinkle the pecan nuts over the plums, divide into 4 portions and serve with the crème fraîche.

rhubarb and banana fool

serves 4

450g/1lb rhubarb, chopped
55g/2oz/⅓ cup brown sugar
2 large bananas, thinly sliced
250g/9oz quark soft cheese

1   Simmer the rhubarb in water until soft, then blend it in a food processor until smooth.
2   When cool, add the sugar and banana to the rhubarb and slowly beat in the quark. Divide into 4 dishes, chill and serve.

tropical fruit salad

serves 4

4 passion fruit, pulp scooped out
425g/15oz can lychees, drained
1 mango, peeled, stoned and cubed
2 bananas, sliced
250ml/9fl oz/1 cup pineapple juice

1   Combine all the ingredients.
2   Divide into 4 dishes and serve.

mango yogurt ice cream

serves 4

2 mangoes, peeled, stoned and chopped
200ml/7fl oz/scant 1 cup semi-skimmed milk
Juice and zest of 2 unwaxed limes
200ml/7fl oz/heaped ¾ cup low-fat bio yogurt
85g/3oz/heaped ⅓ cup fructose sugar

1   Blend the ingredients in a food processor. Pour into a freezer-proof container and put in the bottom of the freezer until the mixture begins to freeze.
2   Turn out into a bowl and whisk, then return to the freezer. Repeat twice more and then freeze overnight. Put the ice cream in the refrigerator for 30 minutes before serving.

resources

Visit

www.naturalhealthguru.co.uk for more information, medical references, and to post questions or comments about the Natural Health Guru programs.

Asthma and allergy

- Allergy UK
  www.allergyuk.org
- Asthma and Allergy Foundation of New Zealand
  www.asthmanz.co.nz
- Asthma Research Online
  www.asthmaresearch.org.au
- Asthma UK
  www.asthma.org.uk
- Australian National Asthma Campaign
  www.nationalasthma.org.au
- European Federation of Allergy and Airway Diseases Patients Association
  www.efanet.org
- European Lung Foundation
  www.european-lung-foundation.org
- Global Initiative for Asthma
  www.ginasthma.com
- World Allergy Organization
  www.worldallergy.org

Complementary medicine associations

- Australian Traditional Medicine Society
  www.atms.com.au
- British Complementary Medicine Association
  www.bcma.co.uk
- New Zealand Natural Medicine Association
  www.nznma.com

- UK Complementary Medical Association
  www.the-cma.org.uk
- UK Institute for Complementary Medicine
  www.i-c-m.org.uk

Aromatherapy

- International Federation of Aromatherapists (Australia)
  www.ifa.org.au
- International Federation of Professional Aromatherapists (UK)
  www.ifparoma.org

Acupuncture

- Australian Acupuncture and Oriental Medicine Alliance
  www.aomalliance.org
- British Acupuncture Council
  www.acupuncture.org.uk
- British Medical Acupuncture Society
  www.medical-acupuncture.co.uk

The Buteyko method

- Buteyko Breathing Association
  www.buteykobreathing.org

Chiropractic

- British Chiropractic Association
  www.chiropractic-uk.co.uk
- Chiropractors Association of Australia
  www.chiropractors.asn.au
- New Zealand Chiropractors Association
  www.chiropractic.org.nz

World Federation of Chiropractic
www.wfc.org

Herbal medicine

International Register of Consultant Herbalists and Homeopaths
www.irch.org

National Herbalists Association of Australia
www.nhaa.org.au

UK National Institute of Medical Herbalists
www.nimh.org.uk

Homeopathy

Australian Homeopathic Association
www.homeopathyoz.org

Faculty of Homeopathy (UK)
www.trusthomeopathy.org

International Register of Consultant Herbalists and Homeopaths
www.irch.org

Naturopathy

Australian Naturopathic Practitioners Association
www.anpa.asn.au

British Naturopathic Association
www.naturopaths.org.uk

Reflexology

Association of Reflexologists (UK)
www.aor.org.uk

British Reflexology Association
www.britreflex.co.uk

Reflexology Association of Australia
www.reflexology.org.au

Quitting smoking

Action on Smoking and Health Australia
www.ashaust.org.au

Action on Smoking and Health NZ
www.ash.org.nz

Action on Smoking and Health UK
www.ash.org.uk

Australian Quit
www.quit.org.au

Quit UK
www.quit.org.uk

Osteopathy

Australian Osteopathic Association
www.osteopathic.com.au

British Osteopathic Association
www.osteopathy.org

Osteopathic Council of New Zealand
www.osteopathiccouncilorg.nz

Yoga

British Wheel of Yoga
www.bwy.org.uk

Yoga Centers Australia
www.yoga-centers-directory.net

index

acknowledgments

The publisher would like to thank the following photographic libraries for permission to reproduce their material. Every care has been taken to trace copyright holders. However, if we have omitted anyone, we apologize and will, if informed, make corrections to any future edition.

page 85 DBP; **93** DBP; **119** Ajax/Zefa/Corbis; **127** DBP; **149** DBP; **155** John Kelly/Getty Images

Height and weight chart on page 67 © Crown copyright material is reproduced with the permission of the Controller of HMSO and Queen's Printer for Scotland.

Author's acknowledgments

I would like to thank my husband, Richard, who willingly provided invaluable back-up and support during those long hours of research and writing. I would also like to thank everyone who has helped in bringing this book to fruition, including Grace Cheetham at Duncan Baird, Judy Barratt and Kesta Desmond – who ensured consistency throughout – and, of course, my inimitable agent, Mandy Little.